How to Succeed at E-learning

How to Succeed at E-learning

Peter Donnelly
Deputy Dean

Joel Benson
Electronic Resources Officer

Paul Kirk
E-Learning Unit Manager

Wales Deanery,
Cardiff, UK

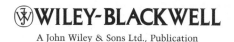

WILEY-BLACKWELL
A John Wiley & Sons Ltd., Publication

BMJ|Books

This edition first published 2012, © 2012 by John Wiley & Sons Ltd.

BMJ Books is an imprint of BMJ Publishing Group Limited, used under licence by Blackwell Publishing which was acquired by John Wiley & Sons in February 2007. Blackwell's publishing programme has been merged with Wiley's global Scientific, Technical and Medical business to form Wiley-Blackwell.

Registered office: John Wiley & Sons, Ltd, The Atrium, Southern Gate, Chichester, West Sussex, PO19 8SQ, UK

Editorial offices: 9600 Garsington Road, Oxford, OX4 2DQ, UK
111 River Street, Hoboken, NJ 07030–5774, USA

For details of our global editorial offices, for customer services and for information about how to apply for permission to reuse the copyright material in this book please see our website at www.wiley.com/wiley-blackwell

Library of Congress Cataloging-in-Publication Data
Donnelly, Peter, 1958–
   How to succeed at e-learning / Peter Donnelly, Joel Benson, Paul Kirk.
      p. ; cm.
   Includes bibliographical references and index.
   ISBN 978-0-470-67023-1 (pbk.)
   I. Kirk, Paul, 1953– II. Benson, Joel, 1969– III. Title.
   [DNLM: 1. Education, Medical–methods. 2. Computer-Assisted Instruction. 3. Education, Distance–methods. 4. Internet. W 18]
   610.71'10285–dc23
                    2012000090

A catalogue record for this book is available from the British Library.

Wiley also publishes its books in a variety of electronic formats. Some content that appears in print may not be available in electronic books.

Set in 9.5/12 pt Minion Regular by Toppan Best-set Premedia Limited
Printed in Singapore by Ho Printing Singapore Pte Ltd

1   2012

Contents

Chapter 9: Looking towards the future, 135

Chapter 10: Conclusion, 143

Acknowledgements

The authors particularly wish to thank our Postgraduate Dean, Professor Derek Gallen, for support, advice and guidance in producing this book. Special thanks also go to Mrs Jo Tucker at Wales Deanery E-Learning Unit, for invaluable support in coordinating many aspects of this work: making amendments, proofreading and liaising with external organisations.

Chapter 1 **Introduction**

The term e-learning can be defined in many ways. In essence, it is about the use of technology to deliver and support learning.

What is this book about? This book is a basic introduction to the world of e-learning.

Who is the book for? This book is pitched at learners and teachers who are considering using e-learning to learn or teach. The focus is on learners and teachers in undergraduate and postgraduate medicine but it will also be useful for all health-related staff.

We have used the term 'teachers' to include undergraduate supervisors, tutors, postgraduate educational supervisors and academic teaching staff.

1.1 Overview of the book

The approach of the book is to provide a framework for learners and teachers to make informed decisions about the use of e-learning and where it fits best. We will identify pitfalls and offer strategies to maximise the use of e-learning. Any views offered are grounded in theory and based on evidence and shared best practice. Examples of some high-quality electronic resources from around the globe are discussed and critiqued.

1.2 Basic issues

To succeed at e-learning, the learner has to succeed at learning. To succeed at e-teaching, the teacher has to succeed at teaching. E-learning should be seen as a tool to enhance the learning experience.

How to Succeed at E-learning, First Edition. Peter Donnelly, Joel Benson, and Paul Kirk.

© 2012 John Wiley & Sons Ltd. Published 2012 by John Wiley & Sons Ltd.

There is a basic question ... is e-learning fundamentally different from any other form of learning? The answer is yes and no. It is qualitatively different in that instead of a sheet of a paper, there is a screen on a PC, laptop or mobile device. The focus of this book is adult learning in healthcare systems in the UK and across the globe. All healthcare systems and professions are increasingly seeking solutions to the challenges of time, finance, culture, ever-changing curricula and geography.

1.3 Challenges as drivers

Particular pressures on adult learners in healthcare communities include the competing demands of the need to maintain clinical, leadership and management skills with the need to continue delivery of the service. Learning in health systems has changed, with less emphasis on traditional educational methods.

Across Europe, including the UK, there have been specific challenges in the postgraduate arena with the implementation of the European Working Time Directive (EWTD) [1] from 1 August 2009 in respect of doctors in training.

With the ever-present need to deliver on-the-job learning in a cost- and time-effective manner, the additional use of technologies to support traditional learning has, at face value, logic. But for institutions and teachers, e-learning developments can be costly in terms of design and development, and also maintenance and appropriately trained staff to support learning.

1.4 The start of technology in learning

There is a view that all e-learning is a form of distance or distributed learning. Distance learning began in earnest with correspondence courses, following the introduction of the Penny Post in 1840.

The use of 'modern' technology, as we now consider it, as an aid to learning had its origins with the invention of the overhead projector (OHP) by Roger Appledorn in the 1960s. The OHP is a good example as it is clear that the technology was not an end in itself but a tool to enhance learning and teaching.

The history of what we now consider basic e-learning tools is recent. The forerunner of the Internet, the Advanced Research Projects Agency Network (ARPAnet), was funded by the United States for military purposes. The ARPAnet was launched in 1969 and paved the way for the development of the World Wide Web by Tim Berners-Lee between 1989 and 1991.

The first email was sent in 1971 by Ray Tomlinson. There is some debate about who first mass-produced the PC and when. The Apple I was launched in 1976, quickly followed by the IBM PC in 1981.

The challenge for health educationists and their learners is to use the current and evolving technology to enhance the learning experience and to ensure it does not become a barrier to learning.

We have had widely used software such as Word and PowerPoint, increasingly sophisticated tools including Personal Digital Assistants (PDAs) and now smart mobile phones. In addition, the Internet has exploded with millions of websites.

One of the key advantages of this is instant access to information. This explosion in accessibility to online and distant electronic resources from around the world is a double-edged sword. There is, however, a need to quality-control information . . . There is now an information overload, or rather an overload of misinformation and an expectation of instant access to information in both our private and working life.

There is an argument that in the early days of e-learning there was less focus on educational pedagogy and that the technology drove the e-learning developments. This has now evolved, whereby most undergraduate and postgraduate learning departments related to health will have active e-learning strategies and use them to deliver and support a range of learning resources.

Not all e-learning is successful, but then neither is all face-to-face learning. As with any learning, effective e-learning has to be underpinned with sound education theory. A sound understanding of how adults learn and how best to facilitate interaction between the learners and the tools (the technologies) is required.

How does one measure success? This is an important question for individual learners, teachers and institutions. We hope this book will help those involved, namely tutors, lecturers, clinical supervisors and their learners, to be better informed of the pitfalls and possible strategies to maximise their learning, including e-learning. Technology continues to evolve at a rapid pace and we hope this book will provide sound principles upon which learners and their teachers can make a judgement regarding the use of e-learning and incorporate it where appropriate into educational programmes and personal study.

If we consider that the first email was sent in 1971, then there has been an explosion in technology in a relatively short period of time and all e-learners and teachers need a framework upon which to base decisions about the use of e-learning. This will be increasingly important going forward. We hope this book is used as a resource to help steer and direct effective e-learning.

Reference

1 NHS Employers European Working Time Directive. http://www.nhsemployers.org/ PlanningYourWorkforce/MedicalWorkforce/EWTD/Pages/EWTD.aspx [accessed on 13 October 2011].

Chapter 2 **E-learning . . . what is it?**

The term electronic learning (e-learning) refers to a range of learning experiences. It is best to view it as a general term, usually used to refer to any use of computers and technology to learn. There are, however, a variety of related terms. In this chapter we will highlight a number of terms used in the field of e-learning and related activities. A broad definition will be offered and examples described where appropriate.

2.1 Definitions

2.1.1 Adobe Flash
Flash is a widely used piece of software that enables you to provide 3D animation and animation of text, drawing and still images. Adobe Flash also supports streaming of audio and video. Alternatives to Adobe Flash are available such as Microsoft Silverlight, (Microsoft's answer to Flash) and Apple's Gianduia, which uses a framework rather than a software approach to provide similar functions.

2.1.2 Adult learning
This includes adult education. Although not specific to e-learning we think it is important to have an understanding of this model.

Adult learning is the practice of teaching and educating adults. A number of adult-learning constructs have been devised, one of which was described by Knowles [1] who first introduced the term andragogy (Greek: 'man-leading'), defining it as 'the art and science of helping adults learn'.

How to Succeed at E-learning, First Edition. Peter Donnelly, Joel Benson, and Paul Kirk.
© 2012 John Wiley & Sons Ltd. Published 2012 by John Wiley & Sons Ltd.

Table 2.1 Knowles' assumptions of adult learners

Assumption	Category
Adults need to know the reason for learning something.	(Need to know)
Experience (including error) provides the basis for learning activities.	(Foundation)
Adults need to be responsible for their decisions on education; involvement in the planning and evaluation of their instruction.	(Self-concept)
Adults are most interested in learning subjects having immediate relevance to their work and/or personal lives.	(Readiness)
Adult learning is problem-centred rather than content-oriented.	(Orientation)
Adults respond better to internal versus external motivators.	(Motivation)

It has also been referred to as andragogy to distinguish it from pedagogy (Greek: 'child-leading'). The essence of andragogy is that as individuals reach adulthood, they come to view themselves as self-directed learners. Knowles described a set of assumptions that have been accepted as more a description of the adult learner rather than as a learning theory. Those assumptions are important to consider in designing and delivering any form of learning and are equally relevant in e-learning (see Table 2.1).

2.1.3 Asynchronous and synchronous methods

Email is the typical example of asynchronous communication. The communications are out of sync in time and place. Advantages include: participants can be in different time zones, less organisation required, flexibility in response and time to reflect. Disadvantages include: lack of continuity, lack of sequence and lack of immediacy.

In synchronous methods, the communications are in real time, such as in chat rooms.

2.1.4 Augmented reality (AR)

Augmented reality is a new blend of technologies that provides applications that add digital artefacts to the real world. These artefacts can be plain text, 3D models or animations, web pages, video or any other digital media type. These artefacts are added to the real world by viewing through a camera and monitor. Some applications, like the example from Audi [2], ask you to print out a piece of paper and hold in front of your webcam. Once the computer detects the paper, it superimposes a 3D animated model of an Audi A1 on the paper. Augmented-reality applications are also available on mobile devices. Acrossair [3] is an augmented-reality browser for the iPhone

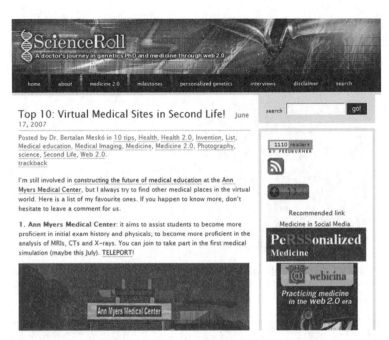

Figure 2.1 ScienceRoll [4]

that allows you to search the Web for a wide range of services close to you. Results are placed on the standard iPhone mapping application when the phone is horizontal. When the phone is held vertically, the camera in the device is activated and the digital information is superimposed over the field of view.

Examples of AR in a health setting (see also Chapter 9):

2.1.5 Avatar
This is a digital 3D persona that is customisable in the virtual world to create your online identity; for example, in Second Life you can become a police officer or a surgeon. This term has been popularised by James Cameron's film of the same name.

2.1.6 Blended learning
This includes hybrid learning.

Heinze and Procter [7] have developed the following definition for blended learning in higher education:

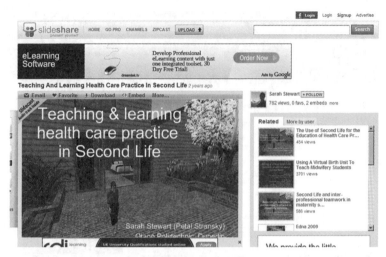

Figure 2.2 Slideshare [5] Reproduced from http://www.slideshare.net/sarahs/teaching-and-learning-health-care-practice-in-second-life © 2012 SlideShare Inc

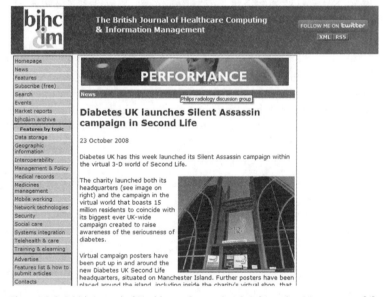

Figure 2.3 British Journal of Healthcare Computing & Information Management [6]

Blended learning is learning that is facilitated by the effective combination of different modes of delivery, models of teaching and styles of learning, and is based on transparent communication amongst all parties involved with a course.

Blended learning refers to the joined-up approach of using online resources to support face-to-face learning. The key is be clear about what can and cannot be used online to support learning. The argument is that clever use of online resources can allow the learners to gain knowledge of the subject prior to face-to-face learning. This can accelerate learning and facilitate more in-depth and focused learning in the face-to-face session.

The decision on whether a learning experience course should be delivered face to face only, online only or as a blended course will depend on the competencies to be achieved, the location and nature of the learner audience and the resources available.

An example of the use of blended learning is the Medical Education MA/PgDip/PgCert. [8] run by the University of Bedfordshire and Hertfordshire Medical School. The programme combines study days, workshops and masterclasses with remote-access online learning.

2.1.7 Blog

A *blog* (a mix of *web and log*) is a type of website where an individual posts comments and pictures and typically shares the day's/week's events. Essentially, a blog is a log of events. Most blogs allow visitors to add comments and hence interact with the blogger and others. Organisations are increasingly using blogs to reflect on key events or hot issues. Most blogs are made up of blocks of text, although some focus on art (art blog), photographs (photoblog), videos (video blogging), music (MP3 blog) and audio (podcasting).

Information on this blog: 'Health Blog offers news and analysis on health and the business of health. The blog is written by Katherine Hobson and includes contributions from staffers at The Wall Street Journal, WSJ.com and Dow Jones Newswires.'

Information on this blog: 'Thoughts, comments, news, and reflections about healthcare IT from Microsoft's worldwide health senior director Bill Crounse, MD, on how information technology can improve healthcare delivery and services around the world.'

2.1.8 Browser plugins

A browser plugin is a small piece of software that extends the functionality of your web browser. Plugins can act as an interface between your browser

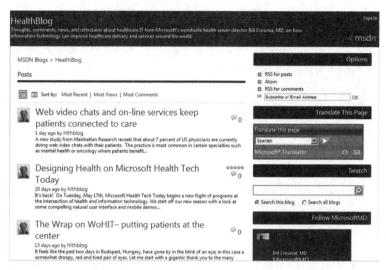

Figure 2.4 HealthBlog [9] Reproduced with permission of MSNBC.com from http://blogs.msdn.com/b/healthblog/, Bill Crounse, MD, © 2011 Microsoft Corporation permission conveyed through Copyright Clearance Center, Inc

and software on your computer, as is the case with the Windows Media Player and Adobe Acrobat plugins. They can also be completely stand-alone as in the case of Adobe Flash Player. In either case, they allow web pages to display content and functions that would otherwise not be available within your browser.

2.1.9 Distance learning

This includes distributed learning (DL) and distance education (DE).

E-learning is sometimes referred to as a form of DL or DE. As defined by Keegan [10], DE involves five qualities that distinguish it from other forms of instruction: (a) the quasi-permanent separation of teacher and learner, (b) the influence of an educational organisation in the planning, preparation and provision of student support, (c) the use of technical media, (d) the provision of two-way communication and (e) the quasi-permanent absence of learning groups. Therefore this is a field of education using teaching methods to deliver learning to an individual or group of learners who are not physically present in what would be considered a traditional classroom, lecture theatre or seminar room.

One characteristic of DE is that the source of information and the learners are separated by both time and distance. Those DE courses that require a physical on-site presence for any reason (including taking examinations) have been referred to as hybrid or blended courses of study.

2.1.10 Electronic course (e-course)

E-courses are courses of instruction that to some extent, either wholly or partially, use e-learning to deliver their content and/or assessments.

2.1.11 E-learning

This includes:

- computer-based training (CBT);
- computer-supported learning (CSL);
- Internet-based training (IBT);
- Web-based training/instruction (WBT/I);
- computer-aided (assisted) learning/instruction (CAL/I);
- technology-enhanced learning (TEL).

E-learning is a generic term encompassing all forms of electronically supported learning and teaching. The *e-* element can be online or not and is best seen as a set of tools to facilitate the learning process. The term is still most likely to be used to describe out-of-classroom and in-classroom educational experiences supported or delivered by technology.

E-learning is essentially computer- and online-enabled transfer of skills and knowledge. E-learning applications and processes include Web-based learning, computer-based learning, virtual classroom opportunities and digital collaboration. Content is delivered via the Internet, intranet/extranet, audio or video tape, satellite TV and CD-ROM. One of the strengths of e-learning is that it facilitates self-paced or instructor-led learning and can include media in the form of text, images, animation, video and audio. The wide range of media available can produce richly interactive learning experiences.

2.1.12 Electronic resource (ER)

ERs are the media building blocks of an e-course. Audio, text, video, animations, Web-based forums and quizzes are examples of media.

2.1.13 Haptic devices

These are devices capable of providing physical sensory feedback to the user and are linked to the computer system (see Chapter 9, page 4 for an example).

2.1.14 Hypertext

Hypertext is electronically linked text. This began as electronic textbooks but has evolved with the Internet. A typical resource is a web page with text and links embedded. These links will take the reader to relevant resources anywhere on the Internet. Hypertext is the underlying concept defining the structure of the World Wide Web, making it an easy-to-use and flexible format to share information over the Internet.

2.1.15 Image files
These are files in different formats that enable you to exchange images, video and animations. Commonly used ones include:
- portable network graphics, PNG (pronounced 'ping') for complex images;
- graphics interchange format, GIF (pronounced 'jiff') for line drawings and simple images;
- joint photographic experts group, JPEG (pronounced 'jay-peg') used for photographs.

2.1.16 Learning management system (LMS)
This is Web-based software that enables trainers to build, structure and deliver e-courses using educational resources of a variety of media on appropriate platforms.

2.1.17 Markup language
A markup language is a modern system for annotating text in a way that is syntactically distinguishable from that text. The idea and terminology evolved from the 'marking up' of manuscripts, i.e. the revision instructions by editors, traditionally written with a blue pencil on authors' manuscripts. Markup is typically omitted from the version of the text that is displayed for end-user consumption. A well-known example of a markup language in widespread use today is HyperText Markup Language (HTML), one of the document formats of the World Wide Web.

2.1.18 Media
Media are the text, images, video, audio, 3D animations or any other visual representations of the message we want to convey to our learners. They are not the structure of the course or the activities it contains; media are the fabric they are made from.

2.1.19 Mobile learning (m-learning)
M-learning is the use of mobile technology to aid learning. Initially we had PDAs and now smartphones and iPads. The advantages include ease of access due to size, just-in-time learning that is easy to achieve, and clinical education at the bedside. These advantages have to be balanced with the cost, accessibility and acceptability. Mobile technology in healthcare settings has gained momentum in the last 5 years, with a number of innovative

approaches, such as the iPhone app iStethoscope that allows you to use the iPhone to measure heartbeat [11] and the top five preferred apps of Harvard medical students as blogged on 19 April 2011:

- Dynamed – Students and physicians rely on this clinical reference tool created by physicians for 'point-of-care' situations.
- Unbound Medicine uCentral – This app serves as a portal of popular medical publications, such as 5-Minute Clinical Consult, A to Z Drug Facts, Drug Interaction Facts, and more.
- VisualDx Mobile – This handy app provides physician-reviewed clinical information along with a huge database of medical images showing detailed variation of diseases.
- Epocrates Essentials – An all-in-one guide to drugs and diseases, this app includes a disease database with conditions, plus photos and details about over-the-counter medications and hundreds of diagnostic and laboratory tests.
- iRadiology – A learning tool for medical students and residents, this app provides quick reviews of classic radiology cases for students to scan during rounds [12].

2.1.20 Multiuser virtual environments

Examples of these environments are:

- Multi-User Dungeon (MUD) – game environments in a fantasy world of fictional races and monsters. Users can explore fantasy worlds, slay monsters and go on predefined adventures.
- Massively multiplayer online role-playing games (MMORPGs) – players are characters in a fantasy world. They control the characters' actions. The game's fantasy world persists over time and is hosted by the game's publisher.
- Second Life (SL) was launched by Linden Lab in 2003 and is basically an online program that allows the development of virtual worlds ('the second parallel virtual life'). Individual participants are called residents (because they reside in the second life) and can interact with each other through avatars. Within the software are the tools to build objects, houses etc. and to interact with them. Because the users can control and develop the infrastructure of the environment (e.g. make a hospital setting), this environment differs significantly from MUD and MMORPGs [4].

2.1.21 Online tutoring

This includes e-moderating, online mentoring and e-tutoring.

Online tutoring refers to the process of tutoring within an online or virtual environment where teachers and learners are separated by time and space. This term also includes online mentoring, e-mentoring or e-tutoring.

Salmon [13] describes the role of the e-moderator as 'promoting human interaction and communication through modelling, conveying and building of knowledge and skills'.

E-moderating can also be provided as part of a stand-alone (un-blended) e-tutoring or e-mentoring arrangement.

An example of this in practice is the Postgraduate Certificate in Medical Education [14] run by the University of Dundee. The course is supported by tutors who are available to answer queries and discuss specific units via email and telephone, with no requirement for the student to attend the physical campus at Dundee. This is a good example of technology supporting the delivery of aspects of the learning experience.

2.1.22 Platform
The platform for text could be a printed page, HTML (web page) or a PDF (Adobe Acrobat), in the same way that platforms for video images could be television, DVD or VHS.

2.1.23 Podcast
A four-part definition of podcast has been described in [15]: a podcast is a digital audio or video file that is episodic; downloadable; program-driven, mainly with a host and/or theme; and convenient, usually via an automated feed with computer software.

So essentially a podcast is . . . a collection of digital media files (either audio or video) that are released episodically. Each episode is usually provided in a format that allows streaming to the device you are using. The difference between formats that support streaming and those that do not is this: a streaming format will allow you to start viewing your video or audio before it has finished downloading. To view a video in a format that does not support streaming you must wait for the entire video file to arrive at your computer before you can view a single frame of it.

The Centers for Disease Control and Prevention host a range of health-related podcasts.

The BMJ also hosts podcasts.

2.1.24 Portable document format (PDF)
A PDF is a standard format for documents that you want to exchange. Each PDF file is underpinned by a standard format including graphics and text.

2.1.25 RSS feeds
The term RSS feed is used to describe a free subscription-based 'push' technology that allows a user to subscribe to newsfeeds sent from a website to

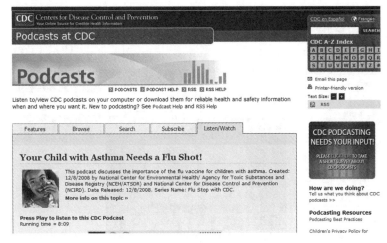

Figure 2.5 Podcasts at CDC [16]

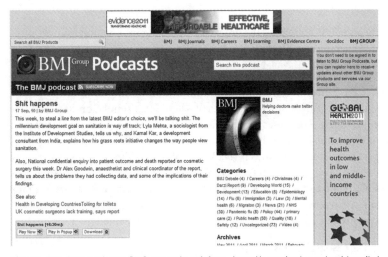

Figure 2.6 BMJ podcasts [17] Reproduced from http://www.bmj.com/multimedia/ 2010/09/17/shit-happens © BMJ Publishing Group Limited 2012

the user's browser. The term is an acronym for really simple syndication. RSS feeds are read using software called an RSS reader. A user can subscribe to a feed by entering the feed's uniform resource locator (URL) into the reader or by clicking a feed icon in a web browser. RSS readers check the user's subscribed feeds regularly for any updates and display the information to

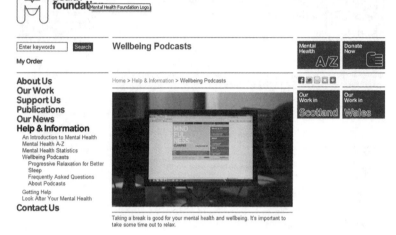

Figure 2.7 Mental Health Foundation podcasts [18]

the user. RSS automates the process of obtaining information from websites in which the user has an interest; any new content is 'pushed' to the browser when it becomes available.

2.1.26 Simulation

With increasing emphasis on patient safety [19], simulation in healthcare education is widely used and has various definitions. The broadest definition of simulation includes the use of a wide range of technologies, from low-tech part simulators to high tech (Da Vinci robotics) to recreate a part or all of the clinical experience. It is this *in vitro* clinical experience, as lifelike as possible, that facilitates and accelerates learning. A wide range of types of simulation have been described [20], some of which involve computer-based systems and e-learning as a strand of the delivery methodology.

2.1.27 Social network sites

These are web sites that focus on providing a service to enable individuals or groups to interact socially. Facebook [21] and Twitter are used worldwide. LinkedIn is the most widely used in the USA. The term social network usually refers to individual-centred services and online community usually refers to group-centred services.

Social sites are increasingly used by organisations to facilitate communication and provide educational material. A wide range of resources are available via these sites, but it is a challenge to identify those that have been quality assured.

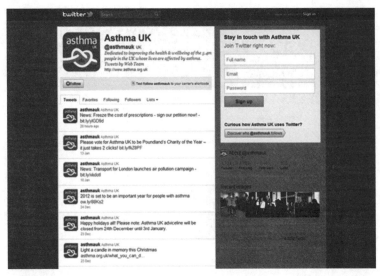

Figure 2.8 Twitter search for asthma [22] Reproduced with permission from Asthma UK twitter.com/asthmauk asthma.org.uk

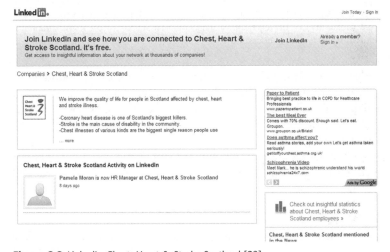

Figure 2.9 LinkedIn Chest, Heart & Stroke Scotland [23]

2.1.28 Virtual learning environment

A virtual learning environment (VLE) is a system designed to support teaching and learning in an educational setting, as distinct from a managed learning environment (MLE), where the focus is on management.

A VLE will normally work over the Internet and provide a collection of tools, such as those for assessment (particularly of types that can be marked

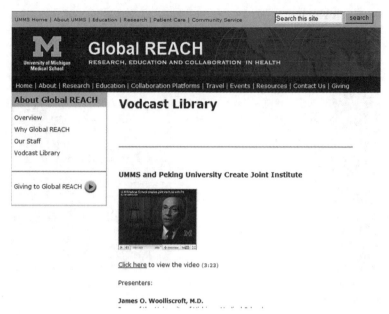

Figure 2.10 University of Michigan Medical School [24] Reproduced with permission from Global REACH, University of Michigan Medical School http://www.med.umich.edu/globalreach/about_vodcast.html. © copyright 2010 Regents of the University of Michigan

automatically, such as multiple choice), communication, uploading of content, return of students' work, peer assessment, administration of student groups, collecting and organising student grades, questionnaires, tracking tools, etc. New features in these systems include wikis, blogs, RSS and 3D virtual learning spaces.

While originally created for distance education, VLEs are now most often used to supplement traditional face-to-face classroom activities – blended learning.

2.1.29 Vodcast
Video podcast (shortened to *vodcast*) is a term used to describe the delivery of video clips on demand. The term is used to differentiate from podcasts, which usually deliver audio.

Vodcasts are used widely in a range of educational settings.

2.1.30 Web 2.0
The term Web 2 refers to the next level of development of software and use of that software on the World Wide Web. A Web 2 site will allow users to

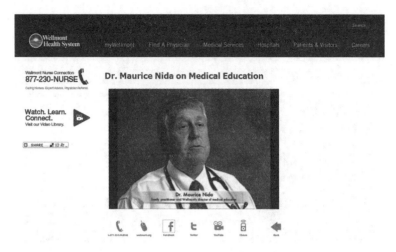

Figure 2.11 Wellmont Health System [25] Reproduced with permission from Wellmont Health System

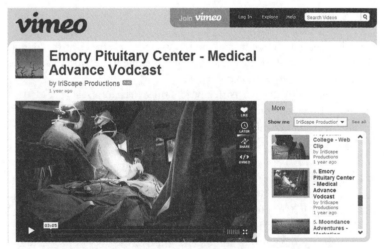

Figure 2.12 Emory Pituitary Center [26] Reproduced from http://vimeo.com/11330915 by IriScape Productions (Iriscape.com) TM + © 2012 Vimeo, LLC

interact with each other in a virtual community. This iterative development has been widely used in health education.

University of Southampton Medical School uses Web 2 to deliver virtual patient scenarios to year 1 medical students. 'Patients' are delivered on a weekly basis and the students explore in their own time; then each is discussed at a face-to-face symposium [27].

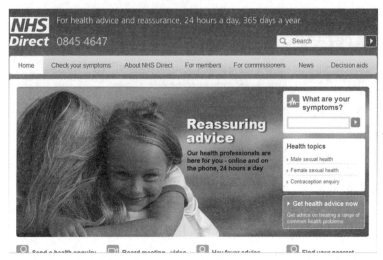

Figure 2.13 NHS Direct [29] © NHS Direct 2012

Michael Barrett, a doctor and clinical associate professor at the Temple University School of Medicine, found that listening to heartbeat audio files drastically improved stethoscope skills.

In a study, 149 doctors correctly identified heartbeats 80 per cent of the time, compared with the usual 40 per cent. Barrett initially distributed his files on CD, until his students suggested he make the files available to iPods [28].

2.1.31 Web browser
A web browser is a software application that acquires presents, formats, and allows navigation of information resources on the World Wide Web.

The commonly used ones are Microsoft's Internet Explorer, Firefox, Safari and Google Chrome. A very common first use of the web browser is to use a search engine to find resources on the World Wide Web; such applications are very large in number and some well-known ones are Google, Yahoo and Bing.

2.1.32 Website
A *website* (also written *web site*) is a collection of web pages containing text, images, diagrams or videos. To be accessible, the website needs to be hosted on a web server linking it to either an internal network or the Internet. The

pages of a website can usually be accessed via a URL. The first page seen when visiting the URL is referred to as the home page. Web pages may be written in any number of programming languages including PHP and ASP. net. When web-browser software makes a request to see a page, the code is executed and constructs a document written in hypertext markup language (HTML). This document contains text and embedded links to media, images and formatting instructions. A language called Javascript is often used on the client side (i.e. the user's computer) to handle interactions such as clicking buttons and filling in forms.

All publicly accessible websites collectively constitute the World Wide Web (WWW). Some sites are open to all, while others require authorisation or subscription to access some or all of the content.

Open sites
One example of an open site is NHS Direct.

NHS Direct's vision as stated is:

> *To be the national healthline, providing expert health advice, information and reassurance, using our world class telephone service and website, and to be the NHS' provider of choice for telephone and digitally delivered health services.*

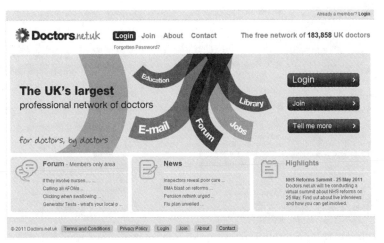

Figure 2.14 doctors.net.uk [30]

Authorised sites

Doctors.net.uk is accessible to all doctors and medical students in the UK and requires a GMC number or medical school and course details (for medical students) to gain membership. The site provides a range of continuing professional development learning experiences.

Other authorised sites to visit include American Academy of Family Physicians [31] and Asian Ophthalmology [32].

2.1.33 What you see is what you get (WYSIWYG) text editor

A WYSIWYG text editor is a simple system that allows you to edit text on wikis or other web pages. Its advantage is that you do not need knowledge of a markup language as the system allows changes in the layout of the text as you edit.

2.1.34 Wiki

A *wiki* is the Hawaiian word for 'fast'. Wikipedia defines a wiki as:

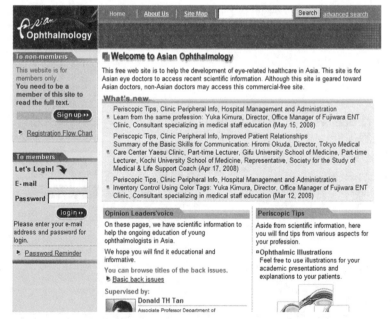

Figure 2.15 Asian Ophthalmology Reproduced from https://www.asian-ophthalmology.com/index.jsp. Copyright 2003, Santen Pharmaceutical Co., Ltd

a website that allows the creation and editing of any number of interlinked web pages via a web browser using a simplified mark up language or a WYSIWYG text editor.

Wikis are used to facilitate and support collaborative work. They are useful in an educational setting as individuals can contribute at their own pace. Wikis can be used in different settings with a range of access and editing rights. Open wikis are essentially open books where anyone can contribute. Other wikis restrict editing rights to preordained groups.

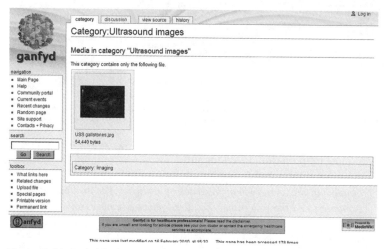

Figure 2.16 Ganfyd [33] Reproduced from http://www.ganfyd.org/index.php?title=Main_Page

---

Box 2.1 Examples of wikis in action

Ganfyd is a free medical knowledge base open to all. It was created in 2005 by a group of doctors and medical students. Only registered medical practitioners or persons working under their direction and a small number of invited non-medical specialists may edit Ganfyd articles. The intention is to make the articles reliable enough for professional medical use. An audit trail is publicly available for each article. Registration is by a variety of mechanisms including a GMC Certificate or equivalent. Ganfyd is described as an evolving textbook of medicine. By October 2010, there were over 2000 page hits a day and it had reached 7000 topic pages with over double that number of pages. This model has subsequently been copied by other medical wikis such as Medpedia.

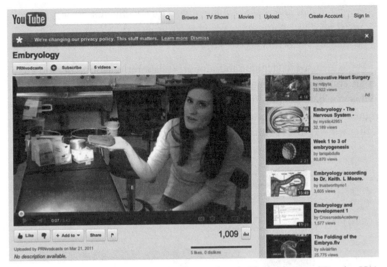

Figure 2.17 YouTube – Embryology [34] Reproduced with permission of Dundee PRN, University of Dundee School of Medicine http://www.dundee.ac.uk/medschool/

A quote from the authors on the site:

> *Simply put this is an evolving textbook of medicine. The medium – computers and the Web rather than dead paper – removes some limitations on conventional text, or reference books and we are taking advantage of that. Perhaps it will help doctors decide what is important, certainly we would encourage contributors to try to distil out issues where other media may be badly out of date or specialisation has resulted in a massive literature of little relevance to most patients.*

2.1.35 YouTube

YouTube is a website that enables users to share video clips. It was set up in 2005 with the purpose of allowing individuals to share video, but it is now used by many organisations via the YouTube partnership programme. YouTube has an increasing footprint of useful educational resources.

2.2 Advantages of e-learning

There has been unprecedented growth in the availability of e-learning opportunities provided by various institutions. There are more and more electronic resources available. All health-service clinicians suffer with

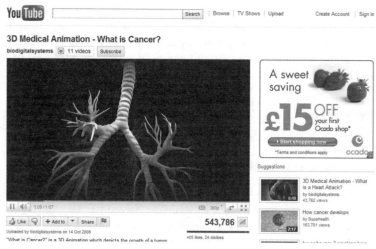

Figure 2.18 YouTube 3D animation – What is cancer? [35] © 2012 BioDigital Systems (www.biodigital.com)

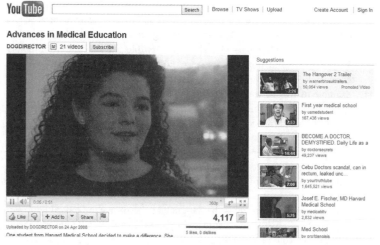

Figure 2.19 YouTube – Advances in medical education [36] Reproduced with permission of Physicians Committee for Responsible Medicine http://www.pcrm.org/

'information overload'. It is not just that they are overwhelmed by the availability of information in general, but also the availability of an excess of information that is relevant to their day-to-day practice. How does a doctor in training, a busy nurse or specialist know which sites are quality assured and fit for purpose?

References

1   Knowles MS. The Modern Practice of Adult Education: from pedagogy to andragogy. Second edition. Cambridge Books, New York, 1980.
2   A1 Augmented Reality.Audi.co.uk.http://www.audi.co.uk/new-cars/a1/a1/augmented-reality.html.
3   Apple iPhone Development. http://www.acrossair.com/.
4   Example of a multiuser virtual environment – Second Life. http://scienceroll.com/2007/06/17/top-10-virtual-medical-sites-in-second-life/.
5   Teaching and Learning Healthcare Practice in Second Life. http://www.slideshare.net/sarahs/teaching-and-learning-health-care-practice-in-second-life.
6   Example of AR in a health setting – British Journal of Healthcare Computing. http://www.bj-hc.co.uk/archive/news/2008/n810041.htm.
7   Heinze A, Procter C. Reflections on the use of blended learning. education in a changing environment. University of Salford, Salford, Education Development Unit, 2004. http://www.ece.salford.ac.uk/proceedings/papers/ah_04.rtf.
8   An example of the use of blended learning – Medical Education MA/PgDip/PgCert run by the University of Bedfordshire and Hertfordshire Medical School. http://www.faculty.londondeanery.ac.uk/programmes/medical-education-MA.
9   Example of a health blog – MSDN blogs. http://blogs.msdn.com/b/healthblog/.
10 Keegan D. Foundations of Distance Education. Third edition. Routledge, London, 1996.
11 Example of mobile learning technology – Upside Learning blog. http://www.upsidelearning.com/blog/index.php/2010/09/13/mobile-learning-innovation-lookup-to-healthcare-for-inspiration/.
12 The top five preferred apps of Harvard medical students as blogged on 19 April 2011.http://www.independent.co.uk/life-style/health-and-families/whats-hot-at-harvard-five-apps-med-students-are-buzzing-about-2270909.html.
13 Salmon G. E-moderating: The key to teaching and learning online. Kogan Page, London, 2000.
14 Example of online tutoring – the Postgraduate Certificate in Medical Education run by the University of Dundee. http://www.dundee.ac.uk/meded/courses/awardbearingcourses/cert-me/.
15 Gil de Zúñiga H, Veenstra A, Vraga, E, Shah D. Digital democracy: reimagining pathways to political participation. Journal of Information Technology & Politics 2010;7(1):36–51.
16 Example of a health-related podcast – Centers for Disease Control and Prevention. http://www2c.cdc.gov/podcasts/.

17 Example of a health-related podcast – BMJ Group. http://podcasts.bmj.com/bmj/2010/09/17/shit-happens/.

18 Example of a health-related podcast – Wellbeing podcasts from the Mental Health Foundation. http://www.mentalhealth.org.uk/help-information/podcasts/.

19 Leape LL. Error in medicine. Journal of the American Medical Association 1994;272:1851–7.

20 Ker J, Bradley P. Simulation in medical education. In: Swanwick T (ed), Understanding Medical Education. Evidence, Theory and Practice. Wiley-Blackwell, 2010.

21 Example of a social network site (Facebook) being used by an organisation to facilitate communication. http://www.facebook.com/diabetesuk?v=wall.

22 Example of a social network site (Twitter) being used by an organisation to facilitate communication. http://twitter.com/#!/asthmauk.

23 Example of a social network site (LinkedIn) being used by an organisation to facilitate communication. http://www.linkedin.com/company/chest-heart-&-stroke-scotland.

24 Example of vodcasts used in an educational setting – University of Michigan Medical School. http://www.med.umich.edu/globalreach/about_vodcast.html.

25 Example of vodcasts used in an educational setting – Wellmont Health System. http://www.wellmont.org/general.aspx?id=1333.

26 Example of vodcasts used in an educational setting – Medical advance vodcast on Vimeo. http://vimeo.com/11330915.

27 Use of Web 2 to deliver virtual patient scenarios to year 1 medical students – University of Southampton Medical School. Choi S, Webb A, Heyworth J, Golestani F, Slaght S. Virtual patients; year 1. 01 Summer 2010:19–20. http://www.medev.ac.uk/static/uploads/resources/01_newsletter/0122_lo_res.pdf.

28 Example of use of Web 2 for heartbeat audio files, CNET News. http://news.cnet.com/Web-2.0-Big-app-on-campus/2100-1032_3-6199687.html.

29 Example of an open website, NHS Direct. http://www.nhsdirect.nhs.uk/.

30 Example of an authorised website, Doctors.net. http://www.doctors.net.uk/.

31 Example of an authorised website, American Academy of Family Physicians. http://www.aafp.org/online/en/home.html.

32 Example of an authorised website, Asian Ophthalmology. https://www.asian-ophthalmology.com/index.jsp.

33 Example of wikis in action – Ganfyd '. . . an evolving textbook of medicine'. http://www.ganfyd.org/index.php?title=Main_Page.

34 Example of educational resources on YouTube. http://www.youtube.com/watch?v=iQBDoOfhKS0.

35 Example of educational resources on YouTube. http://www.youtube.com/watch?v=LEpTTolebqo&feature=related.

36 Example of educational resources on YouTube. http://www.youtube.com/watch?v=FXWqE-wMbT4&feature=related.

[All links last accessed on 14 October 2011.]

Chapter 3 **Evidence e-learning works**

Does it work? Is it effective? These are the common questions asked of all types of e-learning. In this chapter we will explore some of the systematic reviews published in this area and will also focus on subject- and professional-specific examples.

3.1 Systematic reviews

A number of systematic reviews have been published which have reported on the effectiveness of a variety of e-learning and online simulations across healthcare and educational settings. The review articles span computer-aided instruction (CAI), Web-based learning (WBL) and e-learning. Published articles of CAI began in the 1960s [1] and moved to WBL and e-learning with technological advances.

Adler & Johnson [1] conducted a literature review searching MEDLINE and ERIC databases from 1966 to 1998 on CAI as it related to medical education. The aim was to quantify proportions of articles published. The search yielded 2840 citations and 1071 were included for analysis. Three areas were identified; 60% were demonstrations of a CAI application, 11% were media-comparative studies, and 13% were analyses of the CAI field. Of the latter articles, only 1% compared CAI against other CAI studies. The majority of studies were descriptive rather than evaluative. The authors concluded that future research needed to address the following areas: comparison of different CAI methods, economic analysis, curricular development and analysis of CAI in different learning settings, rather than continuing to publish descriptive studies.

How to Succeed at E-learning, First Edition. Peter Donnelly, Joel Benson, and Paul Kirk.
© 2012 John Wiley & Sons Ltd. Published 2012 by John Wiley & Sons Ltd.

Chumley-Jones [2] conducted a review of WBL literature from 1966 to 2002 using Webline and ERIC databases. Of the 206 articles identified, 76 met study criteria and of those 41 (59%) were classified as descriptive and 35 (46%) as evaluative. Authors classified the 35 evaluative studies into four domains:

1 knowledge gain;
2 learner attitude;
3 learner efficiency;
4 programme cost.

Of the 20 studies evaluating knowledge gain, WBL studies were said to report higher post-test scores on multiple-choice tests but overall did not lead to improvements in knowledge in comparison to traditional teaching methods. Of the 31 studies reporting learners' attitudes to WBL, 2 studies showed a preference for WBL over text-based materials; however, authors noted methodological limitations and recruitment bias in the majority of published studies. Predictors of user satisfaction included website accessibility, navigation, attractiveness and download speed. Download speed was identified as a strong barrier to use across allied health professionals.

The authors concluded that it is unclear whether WBL outperforms other media in enhancing learning. Published results varied considerably across users groups and educational level, but published studies suggest there is strong evidence that well-designed WBL programs can improve learners' confidence.

Two studies evaluated changes in efficiency of learning. One study evaluated the cost of WBL. Overall, authors concluded by saying that WBL 'is a valuable addition to our educational armoury, but it does not replace traditional methods such as text, lectures, small-group discussion or problem-based learning'.

Bernard et al. [3] conducted a meta-analysis of the comparative DE literature between 1985 and 2002. The report identified 232 studies. Five quantitative analyses specifically related to DE have been published. Authors concluded overall that many applications of DE outperform their classroom counterparts and that many perform more poorly.

Wutoh et al. [4] conducted a literature search on the effect of Internet-based continuing medical education (CME) interventions on physician performance and healthcare outcomes. Databases searched included MEDLINE, CINAHL and ACP Journal Club and the Cochrane Database of Systematic Reviews. Studies were included if they met the following criteria: randomised controlled trials of Internet-based education in which participants were practising healthcare professionals or health professionals in training. Sixteen studies met the eligibility criteria with six studies showing positive changes in participant knowledge over traditional formats and three studies showing a positive change in practices. The remaining seven studies showed no difference in knowledge levels between Internet-based interventions and traditional formats for CME. The authors concluded that Internet-based CME programmes are just as effective in imparting knowledge as traditional formats of CME but that little is known as to whether these positive changes in knowledge are translated into changes in practice.

Childs *et al.* [5] conducted a systematic review of the literature on barriers to and solutions for e-learning in the health field. The systematic review undertaken included a search of the following databases: AMED (allied and alternative medicine); ASSIA (applied social sciences); CINAHL (nursing and allied health); ERIC (education); HMIC (health management); LISA (library and information science); PUBMED (MEDLINE) and Web of Science (Social Science Citation Index). Authors used the following search strategy: phrases 'e-learning' or 'computer-assisted instruction', limited by the terms 'health' and 'barriers'. From the published literature 142 articles were identified, and a further 19 from grey material yielded a total of 161 articles, 57 of which were included in the final analysis. Inclusion criteria: articles that discussed barriers to and solutions/critical success factors for e-learning in the health field.

In summary, the main barriers to e-learning identified included: requirement for change; costs; poorly designed packages; inadequate technology; lack of skills; need for a component of face-to-face teaching; time-intensive nature of e-learning and computer anxiety. The authors offered the following solutions: standardisation; funding; integration of e-learning into the curriculum; blended teaching; user-friendly packages; access to technology; skills training; support; employers paying e-learning costs and dedicated work time for faculty to deliver e-learning.

Silveira *et al.* [6] conducted a systematic review of published articles in PUBMED and Scopus databases of journals 'measuring the impact of e-learning in the medical postgraduating population'. The authors addressed the following questions:

- How often is e-learning used by medical students?
- What are its effects in learning?
- Is e-learning effective?
- What are the participants' attitudes?

They reviewed 225 articles and found the majority of published journal articles were American studies (45%). No article was found presenting information about the number of medical doctors using WBL platforms or participating in online courses. Of students/practitioners that used WBL, studies reported that they were capable of responding faster and more appropriately versus a conventional course. Six studies reported a general tendency of participants to demonstrate a positive opinion about WBL [7–12]. Two articles identified negative attitudes towards WBL [11,13].

Issenberg *et al.* [14] conducted a systematic review of simulation literature from 1969 to 2003, including peer-reviewed publications in ERIC, MEDLINE, PsycINFO, Web of Science and Timelit, and reports in the unpublished literature that addressed the question:

> *What are the features and uses of high-fidelity medical simulations that lead to most effective learning?*

Of the 607 articles identified, 109 were selected for inclusion. The study concluded that evidence reported suggests high-fidelity medical simulations are educationally effective and simulation-based education complements medical education in patient-care settings. Evidence suggests that high-fidelity medical simulations facilitate learning under the right conditions.

The key findings were the importance of:

- educational feedback 51 (47%) of studies;
- repetitive practice 43 (39%);
- integration into the curriculum 27 (25%);
- range of task difficulty 15 (14%).

Cook [15], in a literature review of WBL using MEDLINE database 2005, identified 115 original articles, and 98 articles evaluated educational technology's use as an instructional tool (descriptive pieces, evaluation studies, research trials and correlational analyses). Cook concluded that:

> *WBL courses usually improve knowledge, and sometimes improve skills, compared with no intervention. Second, WBL courses are usually as good as traditional courses, and one study (Cook [16]) found WBL to be more efficient.*

Cook advised future studies to avoid description of content unless there was a novel approach and that it was not useful to compare WBL against one other medium. He also advised reviewing the cost-effectiveness of WBL, including cost analysis of time, monetary costs and trade-offs. He flagged up key questions such as: What instructional methods are effective in WBL and for what learning outcomes? What makes a simulation (e.g. virtual patients) effective?

Sitzman *et al.* [17] conducted a meta-analysis to examine the effectiveness of Web-based instruction (WBI) compared to classroom instruction (CI) and to examine moderators of the comparative effectiveness. Overall results indicated WBI was 6% more effective than CI for teaching declarative (descriptive) knowledge, the two methods were equally effective for teaching procedural knowledge, and trainees were equally satisfied with WBI and CI. However, when the same instructional methods were used, WBI and CI were equally effective for teaching declarative knowledge. Finally, WBI was 19% more effective than CI for teaching declarative knowledge when Web-based trainees were provided with control (self-paced), in long courses, and when trainees practised the training material and received feedback during training.

Means et al. [18] conducted a systematic review of online learning literature relating to learners between 1996 and 2008. Databases searched included ERIC, PsycINFO, PUBMED, ABI INFORM and UMI Pro Quest. Of 1132 studies identified, 51 articles which met study criteria were included for meta-analysis. The most common subject matter was medicine or health care. The criteria stated studies must compare online learning intervention or blended learning intervention against control group, face-to-face learning and include outcome measures. The results showed that in 11/51 studies, learning outcomes for students learning online compared to a solely face-to-face learning situation were statistically significantly better. In contrast, two studies reported a positive effect for face-to-face learning. Therefore the authors advised caution in the interpretation of the findings, stating that differences may be related to variation in factors other than delivery mode; for example, time spent learning online, course materials and approach.

3.2 Examples of subject-specific studies (categorised by profession)

3.2.1 Healthcare professionals

Pearce-Smith [19] conducted a randomised controlled trial of 17 health professionals with the following objective:

> . . . to establish whether there is a significant difference in terms of knowledge and skills, between self-directed learning using a Web-based resource compared with a classroom-based interactive workshop, for teaching health professionals how to search.

The outcomes measured in the study were knowledge of databases and study designs, and search skills. No significant differences in knowledge of databases and study design, or search skills were reported.

Casebeer et al. [20] conducted a controlled trial to measure the effectiveness of a group of 48 Internet CME activities. Assessment was via case vignette self-assessment questions, administered to US physicians immediately following participation, and to a representative control group of non-participant physicians. Responses to case vignettes were analysed based on evidence presented in the content of CME activities. The results showed that physicians who participated in selected Internet CME activities were more likely to make evidence-based clinical choices than non-participants in response to clinical case vignettes. The authors concluded that 'Internet CME activities show promise in offering a searchable, credible, available on demand, high-impact source of CME for physicians'.

3.2.2 Occupational physicians

Hugenholtz *et al.* [21], Amsterdam University, evaluated the effect of e-learning on knowledge of mental health issues compared to lecture-based learning in a CME programme for occupational physicians (OP). A randomised controlled trial was conducted. Knowledge was tested before and after an educational session with either e-learning or lecture-based learning (both groups n = 35). Results in both groups showed a significant gain in knowledge of mental health care with no significant difference between the two approaches. The results showed there was no significant difference between the experimental and the control group, i.e. e-learning was just as effective as the traditional lecture-based learning within the context of CME and an occupational health setting.

3.2.3 Dental students

Meckfessel *et al.* [22] undertook a comparison study of undergraduate dental students. The experimental group had access to electronic resources compared to the control group who only had traditional lectures. The total sample size was 138 with 71 in the experimental group and 67 in the control group. They compared performance on an end-of-term examination, which was made up of 20 multiple-choice questions (MCQs) with a pass mark of 60%. Using satisfaction questionnaires, they showed that the experimental group had a positive attitude to the electronic resources and that over a 2-year period the failure rate fell from 40 to 2%.

3.2.4 Medical students

Gormley *et al.* [23] undertook a study in Queen's University Medical School with undergraduate medical students. This was essentially a questionnaire in regard to the perceived level of IT ability and accessibility and also experience and attitude towards e-learning. The sample size was 269. The result showed that the students described there being a value in e-learning, but utilisation and accessibility were variable.

Moreno-Ger *et al.* [24] described a study of undergraduate medical students in Spain. The task for the learners was essentially to take a measure of haematocrit. The experimental group (n = 66) played with simulation resources one week before the lab session. The control group (n = 77) did no simulation. The evaluation included a survey measuring the learners' perception of the difficulty of the exercise and a comparison made on the haematocrit values obtained by each learner. The results showed the perceived difficulty of the task was lower with the experimental group (p = 0.16). The haematocrit showed lower dispersion within the experimental group, suggesting higher reliability, and 80% stated that they had a good or very good attitude to e-learning.

Helms *et al.* [25] Wisconsin Medical College, USA, described a comparison study with undergraduate medical students. The topic was the psychosocial aspects of neurology and dementia. The experimental group (n = 66) had access to e-modules on the psycho-social aspects of neurology and dementia. The control group did not have access to the e-modules. The assessments were a written examination via MCQs and an objective-structured clinical examination (OSCE) type of assessment with two standardised patients. The results showed the experimental group had significantly higher scores on the standardised patients but no significant difference for knowledge acquisition on the MCQs.

Romanov and Nevgi [26], Finland, described an uncontrolled study with 3rd-year undergrad medical students. There were 121 participants and the subject area was medical informatics. There were six e-modules with video clips, with a course exam following. The results show that two-thirds of the subjects viewed two or more videos and there was no association between video watching and self-test scores. There was an association, but not a statistically significant association, between video watching and better overall course grades.

Schilling *et al.* [27], Boston, USA, described a study with undergraduate medical students. The subject area was family medicine and associated evidence-based medicine. The experimental group had 134 and the control group 104 participants. The course researched was a 6-week family medical clerkship. Both groups had traditional lecture-based learning and the experimental group had the addition of online modules. The experimental group outperformed the control group and also self-reported more confidence in their understanding of evidence-based medicine within this area.

3.2.5 Postgraduate medical trainees

A pan-European group has published a number of studies comparing e-learning to traditional methodologies of delivery. Hadley *et al.* [28] undertook a study of foundation and internship-level postgraduate medical trainees in the West Midlands, UK, and a number of European sites. The experimental group consisted of 88 and the control group of 72. This was a comparison of e-learning versus lecture-based interventions with knowledge assessment via MCQs. The results showed that the e-learning course was as effective in evidence-based medicine in improving knowledge.

The same group reported a study of postgraduate obstetric gynaecology trainees in six obstetric departments [29]. The experimental group (n = 22) consisted of an integrated e-learning course with the control group (n = 33) having exposure to a traditional lecture-based course. There was a pre and post knowledge assessment via MCQ. The results show the experimental group had slightly higher scores for knowledge gain but this was not statistically significant. Attitudinal changes were similar in both groups.

3.2.6 Dental hygiene

Garland [30], Idaho University, USA, described a comparison of e-learning versus traditional class learning in infection control with 1st-year dental hygiene students. The experimental group comprised 22 and the control group 26 participants. The assessments were at two levels: knowledge acquisition via MCQs and clinical examination similar to an OSCE. The results showed knowledge acquisition was statistically significantly better with the experimental group (p = 0.11).

3.2.7 Primary care

Robson [31] undertook a study in Scotland of primary care physicians (GPs). The subject area was clinical guidelines. The methodology included the use of modified problem-based learning (PBL) e-learning modules and the replacement of the traditional face-to-face group discussion with online interaction. There were 45 participants. The evaluation comprised pre and post knowledge acquisition tested via multiple-choice questions and the results showed no change between pre and post. The subjects were also asked their intention to change practice and this was evaluated by semi-structured interviews of 10 of the subjects, 3 to 6 months after the modules were completed. The results indicated a stated intention to change practice as a result of the e-learning.

3.3 Summary of findings

From the studies described above, general themes have emerged:
- E-learning is equally effective in knowledge transfer and acquisition as compared to traditional methods.
- There is an emerging group who prefer e-learning as a methodology.
- Barriers to e-learning include access, navigation and download speed.

- Well-designed e-learning programmes can improve learners' confidence.
- E-learning is seen as a complementary delivery method with its own unique advantages.
- Electronic environments uniquely facilitate collaborative learning.

3.4 Conclusion

Norman [32], in an editorial on advances in health science education, argues in favour of e-learning being more efficient. The background to his argument is that there is little evidence that different curricula lead to measurably different outcomes [33]. The evidence is that teacher effects are small, accounting for perhaps 7% of the variants, but curriculum effects are even smaller. He also argues that in high-stakes outcomes, for example final exams, there is little evidence that the curriculum has any impact whatsoever. He argues that in fact learners, in this case undergrad medical students, will do whatever is necessary to achieve a desired level of proficiency, regardless of what curriculum they are being taught. He argues that in fact a hidden, very important effect may be the amount of time available to study and therefore if one curriculum or course is more time-efficient, it is likely to be more efficient, although no more effective than another. This background leads on to him arguing that the strength of e-learning and related methods is that it can lead to substantial gains in efficiency and his summary is encapsulated in the following statement:

> *The right research question may no longer be 'Is e-learning more effective than lecture/book/blackboard?' But 'for what kinds of learning is e-learning more efficient and/or effective than other formats?'*

Reviewers generally concluded that caution must be taken as published studies do not effectively assess all factors affecting learning outcomes.

References

1 Adler MD, Johnson KB. Quantifying the literature of computer-aided instruction in medical education. *Academic Medicine* 2000;75:1025–1028.

2 Chumley-Jones HS, Dobbie A, Alford CL. Web-based learning: sound educational method or hype? A review of the evaluation literature. *Academic Medicine* 2002;77(10):86–93.

3 Bernard RM, Abrami PC, Lou Y, Borokhovski E, Wade A, Wozney L, Wallet PA, Fiset M, Huang B. How does distance education compare with classroom instruction? A meta-analysis of the empirical literature. *Review of Educational Research* 2004;74(3):379–439.

4 Wutoh R, Boren SA, Balas EA. eLearning: A review of internet-based continuing medical education. The Journal Continuing Education in the Health Professions 2004;24:20–30.

5 Childs S, Blenkinsopp E. Hall A, Walton G. Effective e-learning for health professionals and students – barriers and their solutions. A systematic review of the literature – findings from the HeXL project. Health Information and Libraries 2005;22(2):20–32.

6 Silveira AC, Baptista AST, Quina C, Carvalho FSG. A systematic review on the impact of e-learning for postgraduate medical education. http://medicina. med.up.pt/im/trabalhos06_07/artigos/Turma18/artigo_intromed_final.doc.

7 Wiecha J, Barrie N. Collaborative online learning: a new approach to distance CME. Acad Med. 2002;77(9):928–9.

8 Wiecha JM, Chetty VK, Pollard T, Shaw PF. Web-based versus face-to-face learning of diabetes management: the results of a compartaive trial of educational methods. Fam Med Oct 2006;38(9):647–52.

9 Casebeer L, Allison J, Spettell CM. Designing tailored Web-based instruction to improve practicing physicians' chlamydial screening rates. Acad Med. Sept. 2002; 77(9):929.

10 Ruiz JG, Mintzer MJ, Leipzip RM. The impact of e-learning in medical education. Acad Med. 2006;81(3):207–12.

11 Sargeant J, Curran V, Allen M, Jarvis-Selinger S, Ho K. Facilitating interpersonal interaction and learning online: linking theory and practice. J Contin Educ Health Prof. 2006;26(2):128–36.

12 Harden RM. A new vision for distance learning and continuing medical education. J Contin Educ Health Prof. 2005;25(1):43–51.

13 Dorman T, Carroll C, Parboosingh J. An electronic learning portfolio for reflective continuing professional development. Med Educ. 2002; 36(8):767–9.

14 Issenberg SB, Mcgaghie WC, Petrusa ER, Gordon DL, Scalese RJ. Features and uses of high-fidelity medical simulations that lead to effective learning: a BEME systematic review. Medical Teacher 2005;27(1):10–28.

15 Cook DA. Where are we with Web-based learning in medical education? Medical Teacher 2006;28(7):594–8.

16 Cook DA. Web-based learning: pros, cons and controversies. Clinical Medicine, Journal of the Royal College of Physicians 2007;7(1):37–42.

17 Sitzmann T, Kraiger K, Stewart D, Wisher R. The comparative effectiveness of Web-based and classroom instruction: A meta-analysis. Personnel Psychology 2006;59:623–64.

18 Means et al. Evaluation of Evidence-Based Practices in Online learning: A Meta-Analysis and Review of Online Learning Studies. US Department of Education, 2009. http://repository.alt.ac.uk/629/.

19 Pearce-Smith N. A randomised controlled trial comparing the effect of e-learning, with a taught workshop, on the knowledge and search skills of health professionals. Evidence-based Library and Information Practice 2006;1:3.

20 Casebeer L, Engler S, Bennett N, Irvine M, Sulkes D, DesLauriers M, Zhang S. A controlled trial of the effectiveness of Internet continuing medical education. BMC Medicine 2008;6:37 doi:10.1186/1741-7015-6-37/.

21 Hugenholtz NIR, de Croon EM, Smits PB, van Dijk FJH, Nieuwenhuijsen K. Effectiveness of e-learning in continuing medical education for occupational physicians. Occupational Medicine 2008;58:370–372.

22 Meckfessel S, Stühmer C, Bormann KH, Kupka T, Behrends M, Matthies H, Vaske B, Stiesch M, Gellrich NC, Rücker M. Introduction of e-learning in dental radiology reveals significantly improved results in final examination. J Craniomaxillofac Surg. 2010 May 6. PMID: 20452231.

23 Gormley GJ, Collins K, Boohan M, Bickle IC, Stevenson M. Is there a place for e-learning in clinical skills? A survey of undergraduate medical students' experiences and attitudes. Med Teach. 2009 Jan;31(1):e6–e12.

24 Moreno-Ger P, Torrente J, Bustamante J, Fernández-Manjón B, Comas-Rengifo MD. Application of a low-cost Web-based simulation to improve students' practical skills in medical education. J Med Inform. 2010 Jun;79(6):459–67.

25 Helms A, Denson K, Brown D, Simpson D. One speciality at a time: achieving competency in geriatrics through an e-leaning neurology clerkship module. Acad Med. 2009 Oct;84(10):67–9.

26 Romanov K, Nevgi A. Do medical students watch video clips in E-learning and do these facilitate learning? Med Teach. June 2007;29(5):484–8.

27 Schilling K, Wiecha J, Polineni D, Khalil S. An interactive Web-based curriculum on evidence-based medicine: design and effectiveness. Fam Med. 2006;38(2): 126–32.

28 Hadley J, Kulier R, Zamora J, Coppus SF, Weinbrenner S, Meyerrose B, Decsi T, Horvath AR, Nagy E, Emparanza JI, Arvanitis TN, Burls A, Cabello JB, Kaczor M, Zanrei G, Pierer K, Kunz R, Wilkie V, Wall D, Mol BWJ, Khan KS. Effectiveness of an e-learning course in evidence-based medicine for foundation (internship) training. JR Soc Med 2010 July;103(7):288–94.

29 Kulier R, Coppus SF, Zamora J, Hadley J, Malick S, Das K, Weinbrenner S, Meyerrose B, Decsi T, Horvath AR, Nagy E, Emparanza JI, Arvanitis TN, Burls A, Cabello JB, Kaczor M, Zanrei G, Pierer K, Stawiarz K, Kunz R, Mol BWJ, Khan KS. The effectiveness of a clinically integrated e-learning course in evidence-based medicine: a cluster randomised controlled trial. BMC Med Educ. May 2009;12;9:21.

30 Garland KV. E-learning vs classroom instruction in infection control in a dental hygiene program. Department of Dental Hygiene, Idaho State University, 921 S, 18th Ave., Stop 8048, Pocatello, ID 83209, USA. J Dent Educ. 2010;74(6):637–43. PMID: 20516303 (PUBMED – indexed for MEDLINE).

31 Robson J. Web-based learning strategies in combination with published guidelines to change practice of primary care professionals. Br J Gen Pract. Feb 2009;59(559):104–9.

32 Norman G. Effectiveness, efficiency, and e-learning. Adv in Health Sci Educ. 2008;13:249–51.

33 Colliver J. Effectiveness of problem-based learning curricula: Theory and practice. Acad Med. 2000;75:59–76.

[All links last accessed on 14 October 2011.]

Chapter 4 **Using e-learning to teach**

Teaching in the online or blended domains requires a range of specialist skills, including some level of proficiency in information technology (IT). The good news is that the skills you already have are transferable and we will mention a range of development software available for those with no access to IT specialists and having limited technical skills later in this chapter. Mastering e-learning requires guidance, time and practice. Having said this, you would be wise to enlist specialist help if it is available to you. It may vastly improve your chances of success, especially on more complex e-learning projects.

First you must be aware that there are many pitfalls awaiting anyone developing electronic resources in medical or health education. You may finish developing a resource only to find that someone has published a much higher-quality resource. Another pitfall is purchasing a high-quality resource and discovering that the assessment component is not assessing outcomes in your curriculum.

This chapter aims to provide you with a means to address the most common pitfalls by providing a template for the systematic development and evaluation of electronic resources. This systematic approach is based on a working knowledge of many approaches to course development [1] and has a number of key stages. These include:

- requirement (define your learners', institutional and your own needs from the resource);
- exploration (market research and resources available to you);
- planning (and building a team);
- development (building and delivering your resource);
- evaluation (assessing the quality and effectiveness of your resource).

How to Succeed at E-learning, First Edition. Peter Donnelly, Joel Benson, and Paul Kirk.
© 2012 John Wiley & Sons Ltd. Published 2012 by John Wiley & Sons Ltd.

Once you complete this process, you will embark on a smaller-scale iteration of it to address any issues revealed by your evaluation. This ensures your resource continues to evolve alongside your stakeholders and educational programme; without this cyclic approach to development, your resource will be destined for extinction. We will explore each of these key stages in some detail.

4.1 Requirement

No educational programme or resource exists in isolation; they all exist in the context of the learners' professional development. The implication of this is that every teaching programme in medical or health education implicitly links with the other programmes on the learners' career paths.

Recognising this has a number of implications. The first is that the resource must be explicit in how it relates to other educational programmes or it will not be seen by learners as a valuable part of their professional development. This is an important component for linking in with your learners' extrinsic motivations [2]. The second implication is that we are providing learning in partnership with governing bodies, healthcare providers and other educational institutions and must consider their needs if our resource is going to be relevant and be seen as relevant.

Considering this, it is important to be clear about who your 1) primary, 2) explicit and 3) implicit stakeholders are and to work out what they will need from the resource you have in mind.

4.1.1 The primary stakeholders: your learners

This is the most important stakeholder group and well worth being thoroughly investigated. Their needs must be at the forefront of your mind for most of the planning, development and evaluation stages of resource development. It is easy to fall into the trap of positively evaluating or developing something that would be appropriate for you but may not meet the needs of your learners.

One way to avoid this is to make a brief profile of your learners. Surveying your learners is the ideal way to approach this but may not always be possible. If this is the case, there may be other sources of information available that could be of use. Your institution may have demographic data showing average age, gender or nationality. If your resource is going to be part of a wider educational programme then prerequisites for the wider programme and information about the IT systems already used in the programme may provide vital information. These can inform you about what you can reasonably expect from your learners' previous knowledge and IT skills.

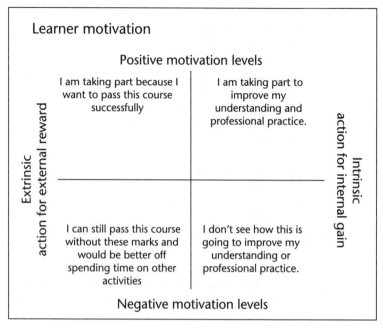

Figure 4.1 Learner motivations

Your profile of them can include:

- *What is their motivation for taking part in your resource?* A motivated learner will put in the effort required to complete your resource successfully. If we are to keep learner motivation high, we must learn a little more about its nature.

If we consider motivation to have a two-dimensional form then we could say that on one axis we have high and low levels of motivation. On the other axis we would have intrinsic and extrinsic motivations. Intrinsic motivations can be seen as the desire to learn, to improve on a personal level. An extrinsic motivation to learn would be completing a course to attain a professional standard.

Intrinsic and extrinsic motivations are not mutually exclusive and coexist quite happily in every learner. For example, an undergraduate medical student will take part in their degree to get a qualification *and* because they want to be a good doctor. However, on specific modules they may want to just get a pass and move on if the topic does not engage them. Reminding them of how the topic contributes to being a good doctor *and* how much it contributes toward their career progression gives you the opportunity to reinforce or even broaden their motivations.

- *What computer programs do they use at work and at home?* Emulating features from computer systems they are already familiar with in your resource has advantages. Emulating these systems where possible reduces redundancy [3] and allows learners to spend less time learning the structure or interface and more time learning course materials. This information also helps gauge IT literacy in your chosen learner group and will be key to developing support structures in the later development phases. If you are evaluating a resource you should consider whether the interface and navigation uses features your learner group will already be familiar with.

- *What kinds of technology do they have access to?* Libraries and work computers may provide access to the Internet but their use is often restricted by security policies or high demand. It may be reasonable to expect some learner groups to own a laptop or desktop PC with broadband connection. Other learner groups may own the latest smartphones. Being aware of the technologies they have access to and any restrictions will help you choose the right technology and create a resource suitable for all your learners.

  If you are evaluating an existing resource, try using it in the same setting you expect your least equipped learner to be accessing it from. This is an important point. Tailoring the technology to the lowest common denominator will reduce disengagement by your learners. It is also useful to be explicit about the specification of technology required by your learners.

- *What formal or informal education have they completed?* This will determine your course prerequisites and decide whether you will need a course structure that takes a variety of learner levels into account. Don't make assumptions about the whole learner group from your own experience.

- *How many hours are they likely to be able to commit; where are those hours likely to be found?* This will have an impact not only on course duration but also on how you structure the instructional materials. If your resource contains medium-sized sections of learning material then your learner will need to find medium-sized time slots to address them. Smaller sections create the option of doing coursework in smaller time slots and make it easier for your learner to find the time to participate.

  Your choice of media can also help learners find the time to take part. If you supply an audio version of written materials then the learner can listen to it on the bus or in the car (if they own an MP3 player).

- *How diverse are they?* Consider how working and personal cultures including attitudes toward technology, their mastery of English and religious beliefs may also play a part in your course design; for example, it may not be wise to schedule an examination on Christmas Day or on Eid. Ramadan may be a stressful time for some learners so this needs to be taken into account when setting deadlines.

- *Are temporal and geographic locations important?* Knowing where your learners already take part in training can be helpful. Expecting them to take part in your training from a location they already train in can provide you with IT and staff resources. It also provides a familiar environment for them.

Knowing if they have the opportunity to learn together or are split by shift patterns or timetables can also have implications for evaluating or designing a resource. If they all know each other well and are used to taking part in group activities offline then online group activities like forums and wikis may produce good results relatively quickly.

The information you gather may produce a mixed picture of learners who are young, old, together and separated. This picture will be of more use if you use the information to create two learner profiles illustrating the extremes that your learner group encompasses. These profiles should also include the features that are common to both groups.

Once you have these profiles, you will be able to ask yourself if the two hypothetical learners would be capable of navigating every aspect of the resource you have in mind. If the answer is yes then your other learners should also be OK.

4.1.2 Explicit stakeholders

These are the stakeholders you have some direct responsibility to. Creating a bullet list with an outline of their needs will be enough for evaluating a resource that already exists. If you are starting afresh then you can use the bullet list later on to draw up a project plan and inform your design decisions. Your explicit stakeholders can include the following.

- *Heads of academic schools, deans of education, and health-service and business managers.* This group may need cost-effective solutions utilising resources (staff time, IT systems) that are not e-resources already in place. Outline the benefits of creating your resource and where it fits in with institutional strategy. If there are possibilities for generating revenue then also outline how this might be achieved and supported.
- *Administrative, support and technical staff.* Will learners using your resource be supported by these staff? If so, outline any changes your resource would make to their support role.
- *Quality assurance and other standards.* Are there any quality standards or policies you must adhere to? Will you be asked to produce specific reports

on pass rates, uptake or other metrics beside assessment results? What are your plans to cater for these needs?

4.1.3 Implicit stakeholders

These are the stakeholders you have no direct responsibility to provide for but explicitly doing so will make it easier for learners to see how your resource fits into their career progression. Not all the needs of your implicit stakeholders will be of interest to your learners and extrinsically motivate them. Despite this, it may still be worth aligning your resource to meet those needs if it can be done without lessening the quality of the educational experience you have planned for your learners. Doing this may lead to those bodies providing support for your efforts. This practical help could include endorsement, expertise, accreditation or even funding.

In the UK, regulatory bodies such as the General Medical Council, General Dental Council, and Nursing and Midwifery Council, and in the USA state regulatory boards, are key implicit stakeholders. Others include the following:

- *Royal colleges, commissions and councils*: does your resource address any of their strategic priorities or map to published curricula?
- *Competing institutions*: competing institutions usually have a large number of shared objectives and similar IT systems. Are there opportunities to share the finished resource if both institutions contribute expertise and resources to building it? If so, you may be able to create a much higher-quality resource than if you were to work in isolation.
- *Pre and post institutions*: how does your resource form the foundation of further learning in your own and other institutions? Does it form a natural next step for learners who may have undertaken previous courses?
- *Healthcare providers*: does the resource meet any corporate needs of healthcare providers (e.g. probity, clinical governance or legislative issues)?

4.1.4 Project scope (your requirement)

We address this now because investigating the needs of your stakeholders may have had an impact on what you need to get from the resource. Breaking your requirement into the following sections will help you to systematically focus on the various aspects of your resource. Once you have completed it for your requirements, you can include and expand on the bullet points created for your stakeholders where appropriate.

You will have then created the basis of a *project scope* to communicate what you have in mind to those who will be helping you build the resource. The scope will also help you keep track of your intentions while the resource develops and help set criteria for determining if the resource has been successful.

A project scope includes:

1 outline;
2 objectives;
3 assessments;
4 integration and communications.

Outline

This is the first section of your scope statement. Here we provide an overview to clarify what the resource is about, why it is needed and what the benefits are for all stakeholders. Remember to address your needs first and move on to other stakeholders.

The clarity this exercise provides will also be invaluable for keeping your project focused. It will also be useful for setting evaluation criteria to determine if any purpose-built resources meet your needs. In your outline provide a brief overview of the topics it will cover and why the resource is needed. It is important to address what gap(s) in the existing range of provisions it fills. This section will also cover what improvement it would or hopes to make for you and other stakeholders.

Objectives

The systematic writing of objectives was first introduced as a way to express the type and depth of learning an assessment was supposed to measure. They are the 'specific, observable, and measurable' outcomes learners are expected to demonstrate after receiving instruction [4]. Using a common framework for defining objectives meant that institutions could share assessments that met specific criteria with some degree of certainty [5 p.212]. The framework devised for this was Bloom's taxonomy of learning [5 p.213], which divided learning into three domains (cognitive, affective and psychomotor), each with a hierarchy of six levels indicating the depth of learning to be demonstrated. The most common domain referred to within online learning is the cognitive domain. The hierarchy for this domain includes:

- knowledge;
- comprehension;
- application;
- analysis;
- synthesis;
- evaluation.

Why should we write these objectives, given that sharing assessments with other institutions may not be our top priority? One answer is that they help us to clarify the outcomes we hope to see and determine whether our assessments actually assess these outcomes. Once we are clear about what our assessment criteria will be, we can determine exactly what instructional material and activities the learner will need in order to be able to satisfy them.

Explicit objectives also serve a purpose for more proactive or independent learners. Having access to the objectives means they can determine and meet their own needs using the instructional materials you have provided and sources of their own. This allows learners to cater for their own learning styles.

One way to approach writing objectives is to use one of the methods suggested by Waller [1]. This involves looking at each objective as a sum of four parts. These parts are:

- action;
- condition;
- standard;
- audience.

The audience and conditions form the first part of our objectives because they usually remain the same. This avoids redundancy [3] and makes your objectives easier to read. The action and standard usually differ for each point. The action lets the learner know what they will be expected to do after they have gone through your instructional material. This directly relates to the hierarchy set out in Bloom's taxonomy of learning. The standard sets out the level of competency required.

Comparing our objectives to those in any resources we may be evaluating can clarify whether they meet our needs.

Assessments

Now the objectives have been set, you can start looking at what assessment strategy would be appropriate for your resource. For the purpose of the scope statement, you will only need to outline an assessment strategy and highlight areas you may need extra help in (like writing the questions and validating the assessment).

At this point it is worth considering that assessment can be seen as lying along a continuum. At one end is formative assessment; this provides detailed feedback for each learner interaction with the aim of helping them to assess their own understanding of existing or new knowledge. This is using assessment as a tool to aid and direct learning activity.

At the other end of the scale is summative assessment, used to observe a change in the learner's behaviour [3] with the aim of determining whether they have achieved the course outcomes.

Sample Objective

On completion, the learner will be able to: orally present a new patient's case in a logical manner, chronologically developing the present illness, summarizing the pertinent positive εt negative findings as well the differential εt plans for further testing εt management.

Anatomy of the Objective

On completion, the learner: Providing the condition and audience part of the objective respectively.

'orally present' and 'summarizing': Actions relating to the 2nd level of the cognitive domain (comprehension).

logical manner, chronologically developing, pertinent positive and negative findings, differential and plans for further testing and management. These all provide information on the standard expected of the learner for this objective.

Figure 4.2 A sample objective and its anatomy

The disadvantage of *formative* assessments is that busy learners may decide not to undertake them because they usually do not count toward their final marks. Learners who adopt this strategy can slow or derail their progress considerably. The disadvantage of *summative* assessment is that it is not intended to provide the detailed feedback necessary to inform further progress with the learner.

A good assessment strategy aims to strike a balance between the formative and summative ends of the scale. The assessments in your strategy should be weighted toward their primary function but it is acceptable to make allowances for the other roles assessment can play. If you decide that your formative assessments cannot play some part in determining completion then many LMSs can be configured to withhold course materials until activities like formative assessments have been completed. Similarly, detailed feedback for summative assessments can be withheld until the examination is closed. The feedback can then be released with the scores or could be used as the basis of a telephone conversation with the learner about their progress and future development (if you had the resources to do so).

The implications of this point for anyone evaluating pre-existing resources are twofold. First, it is important that the resource has an assessment regime that meets your objectives and supports learning. Second, it is important to consider how you will be able to find out which of your learners have completed it. Some resources issue named and dated certificates of completion. Your strategy could be as simple as asking the learner to print or send their certificate to you as evidence.

Integration and communication (with teaching programmes or curricula)
At this point you will have a clear idea of what you are looking to accomplish with your resource and can see where it is likely to fit in with your stakeholder needs (other than your learners). List the needs you would like to address, what you plan to provide and your point of contact with that stakeholder group. A comprehensive communications strategy is key.

4.1.5 Supporting your learners
It is important to identify the learner support systems as there is a connection [6] between support provided and learner completion and satisfaction. It is best to clarify who will provide academic, technical and administrative support and provide a clear definition of each of these roles. The stakeholders you have identified earlier in this document may be willing to help out as they have a vested interest in your learners and the success of your resource. There are four basic types of support necessary in online learning. These are:
- academic (help with the subject matter);
- non-academic (counselling, pastoral support);
- technical (help with the delivery medium);
- administrative (help with enrolling, graduating, funding and other administrative functions).

With each of these it is vital to have a clear plan of action, identifying the type of support, who will provide it, boundaries and any resource implications.

4.1.6 Evaluation
Designing an e-learning resource involves building a picture of the requirement, finding out what you can about your stakeholders and basing the design on that picture. You are never going to start with all the answers and even if that was the case, the design would still be based on what you assume will work with the theory and experience at your disposal. There is nothing wrong with assuming; without it you would never find a way forward, but

you must be aware of where those assumptions have been made and check if they are correct. The more experienced your team is, the more likely their assumptions will be correct. If you do not have a team then it is useful to attempt to enlist the help of critical friends as their views may prove invaluable in revealing the assumptions you didn't realise you had made. Even with these measures, there is only one way to find out whether your assumptions have been correct and your design really works.

If we were to design a face-to-face session on a topic, the first time we delivered it would be about finding out whether the learners were engaged, whether we covered the necessary amount of ground and whether the learners understood (amongst answering other questions). In a face-to-face environment, most of our questions can be answered by observing the learners and getting feedback on short evaluation forms. We would then make a few changes where we felt improvements could be made.

Online learning environments rarely provide us with the same opportunity to observe our learners directly and it is unlikely that we can survey after each activity to test for effectiveness. If we did, then it is possible that the learners would spend more time on surveys than on the learning material. A solution to this problem is to do the following.

- *Get usage data from as many sources as possible*: Google Analytics [7], Piwik [8] and others can go some way to showing when, where and how long people spent accessing your resource. This can provide useful information on how long it takes to complete the online parts of various topics and determine whether you have any problems with navigation. Learning management systems can also provide valuable usage statistics. Any formative assessments in the resource can help you see whether learners struggled with particular concepts. The number and type of requests for support can also reveal areas where learners struggled. Cross-reference your data to see whether the picture gained from one source is supported by another.
- *Target and space your surveys*: add short surveys at regular points through your resource. How many you add will depend on how long it takes to get through the resource itself. If it takes a few hours or days then one may well be enough. If the resource takes an academic year to complete then one per month would be ideal as long as they are short. If they are placed any further apart, it is unlikely that the learner will remember the material being surveyed in too much detail. If there are areas you are unsure about then place surveys directly after them if at all possible. Also bear in mind that surveys need to provide space for feedback on issues beyond those explicitly addressed. After all, you may have overlooked the issue that your

learner would most like to talk about. Ensuring that the survey gives the opportunity for free-text answers is useful.

- *Survey all your stakeholders*: doing this will determine whether your plans do indeed meet their needs or not. It will also help to determine whether their needs have changed.
- *Get professional help*: for your evaluation to address assumptions rather than create more assumptions, it must be based on sound principles.

The next step is working out exactly what you need to evaluate. The challenge we have here is that 'quality' is subjective. What makes a good-quality resource will change depending on who you ask. This means that different stakeholders will be judging the quality of your course using different criteria. For example, the International Standards Organization (ISO) is responsible for setting international standards for everything from car parts to courses. Their view is that quality assurance (QA) is an activity designed 'to establish processes that will maximise service to customers'. Other definitions state QA is a 'proactive, rigorous and ongoing process of planning and self-assessment which will enable (universities) to ensure the quality outcomes expected by their students and the wider community'.

There are a number of models available that try to encapsulate QA. Some of these may be very useful while others may not quite meet your needs. These models vary in a number of ways including:

- the features used in the resource to assess quality;
- the emphasis on self, peer and independent evaluation;
- the target for the model.

Some models are generic and can be applied to quality assuring any product (like the ISO standards). Others are intended to benchmark quality with the aim of internationalising qualifications gained online [9]. Others are for learners to be able to determine for themselves what makes a good-quality resource and are undoubtedly the most useful for anyone developing or evaluating a resource. They also successfully capture the fundamental features that any online course should provide. The list below is loosely based on the features from the learner-centred QA models already mentioned. Some of the points in this list may be covered by the course or programme that your resource fits into. Even so, these points need to be considered if not included on your list of evaluation criteria:

- Can your learners see a sample of the course materials and activities?
- Have arrangements for providing feedback been detailed together with the expected amount?
- Have the entry requirements and level of study been clearly stated?
- Are the types, access routes and response times of support systems clearly shown?

- Have details of offline activity been provided and what type of activity is this (attending a face-to-face session, hours reading or researching)? How much of the final grade does this account for?
- Can the learners talk to former students or see results of course evaluations?
- Have previous students been successful?
- Is the resource/course accredited or recognised by anyone?
- Has any information about your institution or company been provided? This should include who the regulators or external assessors are and any affiliations or partnerships.
- Have complaints and refund policies been detailed?
- How often does evaluation and review take place? Who participates in this (internal, peer or external)?

Here you start reaping the benefits of the hard work and investigation you have (hopefully) already done. You already know who your stakeholders are and what their needs may be. You can add these to your list of evaluation criteria and make a note of the stakeholder it concerns against each one. Your stakeholders will have some shared needs so there will undoubtedly be considerable overlap.

Consider how you can measure each of the criteria on the list. Some measures will be as simple as making sure certain information is available on the resource's home page. These items will contribute toward our course structure and design. Some criteria will be best measured with a survey. Gathering statistical data via surveys is a professional discipline in its own right and beyond the scope of this chapter. We would advise the use of a standard survey that research has already proven to be effective and unbiased. If you have to change one of these to meet your needs then seek professional advice on whether your changes are likely to significantly alter the validity of the survey. If your institution has adopted a QA model, there may be someone in charge of helping you to comply. They may be helpful in creating an unbiased survey that will yield valid results. Don't worry if you cannot put measures against all the criteria right now; you will revisit your criteria throughout the development to fill any gaps.

Before we move on from QA, it is worth noting three aspects of the approach described by Jack Kuomi [10].

The first is that the aim of course development should be to build quality into the resource rather than rely on evaluation to filter bad quality out.

This means you would regularly review development plans and progress with a steering group that represents your stakeholders, subject matter, and technical and support staff. If you do not have access to all these individuals, you will have to make do with whoever is willing to help. This approach is like a sub-implementation of a continuous quality improvement model (CQI).

This approach may extend development time initially but it does mean:

- the developed resource will cause as few problems as possible for the first cohorts;
- the lower-quality aspects will be spotted and addressed sooner, which means the time to delivery of a high-quality resource is actually shortened.

The second point worth noting in Kuomi's approach is the balance between evaluation and improvement. Although Kuomi expresses this in a controversial way, the principle of striking a balance between evaluation and other course development activities is essential if we are to make the most of the time and effort invested by our learners and the course development team.

Another key point is that the purpose of evaluation is to facilitate improvement. This means our QA plans will need to account for the time and people necessary to address any issues revealed by the evaluation.

Now that you have reached this point, you will have an outline and two learner profiles. These documents will prove invaluable for providing the information you need to get support for building your resource. They will also be invaluable for providing the information you need to make the correct design decisions for your learners and other stakeholders and allow you to evaluate existing resources with an informed viewpoint.

4.2 Exploration

At this point you will have a solid understanding of what you need from a resource, whether it is built in-house or by an outside agency. The next step is to find out whether anyone has already developed something similar to the resource you have in mind. A good place to start your exploration is with your favourite search engine. There are also a number of chapters in this book (including Chapter 6) that will point you in the right direction.

If you do find something similar, we would suggest evaluating it using the QA, learner profiles and other documents you have already written. If it does not fulfil all your needs, it may still be possible to use it by adding the missing pieces with an LMS. This would be a portal approach to e-learning and has proved successful for a number of institutions around the world.

4.2.1 Using media in learning

Media, as defined in Chapter 2, are the text, images, videos, audio, 3D animations or any other visual representation of the message you want to convey to your learners. They are not the structure of your course or the activities it contains. The media are the elements that combine to make up the fabric of the learning experience.

Research into appropriate use of media seems contradictory at first glance. Some advocate a learner-centred approach that includes providing instruction in a variety of media to allow for different learning styles [11]. Others warn that providing too much choice confuses the learner and removes the chance for learners to develop their learning styles [4]. We would suggest that providing one appropriate combination of media for your message would be better than providing a variety of media to meet all learner preferences. There is also an argument that providing materials to meet all learner preferences and learning styles is an abdication of the responsibilities of the instructional designer. A major part of that role is to choose the media and activities best suited to the task at hand.

It is likely you will already have experience of listening to audio, watching video, reading web pages and working with text documents. This will give you an idea of the possibilities of each medium for learning, but to make the correct choice you will need to be aware of the other features of each media type.

- Text: the most common and underrated media type available. Formatting pages of text in the same way that chapters are formatted in a book can lead to materials that are hard for learners to engage with. Magazines and newspapers can provide ideas for ways to format text in more engaging ways.

- Video: standards and formats are changing rapidly, and so is the level of skill and equipment needed to produce high-quality video. Be aware that video files are considerably bigger than text or image files. If you plan to make them available on the WWW then make sure the infrastructure you use has the bandwidth available to deliver it successfully. Video will need special browser plugins for it to be viewed (for now at least). Do your learners have access to browsers with these plugins? Has your institution approved and supplied specific plugins for video? Uncoordinated camera movement, bad acting, excessive background movement and bad audio are all likely to distract the learner from the message you are trying to convey. The amount of distraction or static is often the major difference between amateur and professional video productions.

- Audio: the standards and expertise required are changing as rapidly as in video. The issues of distraction, browsers/audio players and audio file sizes also apply to audio production.

- Images: this is a mature technology so format changes are not an issue. All media authoring software and platforms for delivery accept images of one type or another. The different formats available (png, jpg, gif and others) are used to optimise specific image types for specific uses. Photos for web delivery are usually best optimised as jpg, jpeg or png-24 formats. Graphics, diagrams or charts for the Internet are usually optimised best in gif or png-8 formats. Animated images earned a bad reputation through misuse in their first few years of use on the Internet. This prejudice was well deserved but there are times when animated images are a good choice (i.e. demonstrating the rain cycle). Without optimisation, images can cause pages (web and other formats) to load very slowly and again, be likely to cause distraction from the point you are trying to make.

- Interactive media: authoring tools like Adobe Flash allow the creation of working models of objects and systems that can change state depending on learner input. These can be stand-alone applications or viewed in a web browser with a plugin. These take more time and technical skill to produce as they usually involve some degree of programming.

- 3D models and virtual worlds: 3D models can take considerable technical skill to produce, but software is emerging that gives results with the need for much less technical knowledge. Models can also be bought or freely downloaded in a variety of formats. These can be uploaded into Web-based virtual worlds like Second Life (see Chapter 2). However, it is worth bearing in mind that navigating these environments and learning the etiquette of interacting with other users or learners takes time to master. Learners new to this medium must be allowed the time to acclimatise and be supported through this process before they are in a position to focus on the material rather than the mechanics of interaction. How much time is needed depends on your learners' previous experiences with 3D worlds, what you are asking of them and the world you choose.

The best approach to choosing the correct media is to look at each part of the message you want to convey. If one point can be best conveyed with a page of text then use a text-based medium like a basic web page or PDF. If another part of the message would be best illustrated with a diagram then add one at the relevant point. If you need to illustrate repetitive movement or cycles then animation would be the most appropriate choice. If you choose the medium best suited to each individual point in your message, you ensure that the message is heard as clearly as possible. Once you have decided on the appropriate media for each part of your message, you can choose the activities to support learning.

4.2.2 Theories and perspectives on how we learn

In developing resources, it is important to have at least a basic understanding of how we learn. This will help you design the resources in an effective manner. There are a number of schools of thought on how we learn. Each goes some way to explain the mechanics of learning, but none of them provide guidance on every aspect of learning. If we start with an example of learning, we can see how each of the different approaches explains a part of the process and how they can be used together to support learning.

This example is one possible route a child may take through learning to write:

1   A child begins to speak and understand spoken words.
2   A child is introduced to books and is read to by their parents. The parent shows the pictures and words in the book and the child begins to understand that the book contains a story. The child asks for the same book to be read to them repeatedly.
3   The child is introduced to the words that make up the story and can see that the shapes (letters and words) contain more of the story than the pictures.
4   The child has reached a point where their coordination is good enough to form letters. They are introduced to letters and forming written words (usually their own name, 'mum' or 'dad').
5   Spelling and grammar are introduced; skill in reading and speech has progressed alongside their progress with writing, allowing the possibility of self-expression via their new skill (at this stage it may be 'I am three').
6   Schooling starts and progression of their basic written (and other) skills is structured. Their skill in writing is applied more creatively than before and a handwriting style is consciously formed. The child learns to adapt their grammar and spelling to suit short-message digital media (SMS, chat windows and email).
7   Years pass and the child is now an adult with professional qualifications working in medicine. They have mastered the skill of writing and can apply it appropriately in a variety of contexts (i.e. letter to a friend, written academic paper, taking patient notes).
8   Our child now has a 2-year-old of their own and reads books to them.

This example is contrived, but should be good enough to look at how the main theories of learning attempt to explain what is going on here.

Before we look at each of the schools of thought, we must acknowledge the common ground between them. They all maintain:

1   Learning only happens through activity of some sort.
2   Feedback is essential for progression of learning.
    The schools of learning are:
1   behaviourist;
2   cognitivist;
3   constructivist.

There is also a fourth school of thought emerging that can be seen in the perspectives of situationist and connectivist theories. We will visit these theories briefly as they may provide insight for activities and designs that may help you break new ground in e-learning.

Behaviourist school

The behaviourist school is one of the first set of theories of learning and maintains that learning can only be said to have happened when there is an observable change in behaviour [12]. This will only happen if there is activity, response, assessment and feedback that lets the learner know whether their response was the appropriate one. This is a cycle which finishes when the desired response is observed.

In our example, activity and feedback are always present in one form or another. Early on, feedback is given by the parent and then by the teachers in school. As the skill of writing is applied throughout the child's life, others will provide feedback in more subtle ways. The learner eventually starts assessing whether their application of the skill was successful or not and makes changes to the way they apply their skill. This demonstrates a cycle at work, but shows a cycle that does not end at the point where the required response is observed. It also does not explain why the child eventually takes responsibility for development of the skill and continuation of the cycle. This approach does not consider the other skills necessary for the development of writing, like speaking and hand–eye coordination, or the natural progression from learner to teacher we see in this example.

Behaviourist design principles and activities include:

- providing the learner with an idea of what they are expected to achieve (objectives);
- a course structure that starts at basic principles and moves on to activities that allow a display of the behaviour change described in the course objectives;
- assessment at key points in the path provided (formative assessment);
- feedback as close to the assessments as possible.

Cognitivist theory

The cognitive approach [13] was developed in the 1960s and focuses on the actual mechanics of acquiring knowledge. It outlines the duration of our attention span and considers factors that can distract from learning the points in hand. This school also addresses the limitations of short-term, working and long-term memory and has theorised on the optimum conditions for moving information from one type of memory to the other. When something new is learned and moved from working to long-term memory, one of two things happen; either it is added into their existing network of knowledge (assimilation), or any differences between the new and existing knowledge are reconciled and the result is reflected as part addition, part adaption (accommodation) [4 p.10], The amount transferred is dependent on the amount, or depth, of processing that takes place during transfer. It also addresses the phenomenon of automation. This is where a new skill takes large amounts of the learner's mental faculties to perform. After repeated performances of the skill, it takes much less concentration to perform the task. At this point they are capable of reflecting on the finer points of their performance and how it fits in with their environment.

This school also considers individual learning styles and the effect that different personalities can have on the way individuals learn. It categorises personalities and learning styles in a number of ways including abstract conceptualisers and active experimenters, field dependent and field independent assimilators and accommodators.

This theory implies that the act of teaching is to provide material that builds on existing knowledge and to guide interpretation of new information through activities that promote deep learning.

In our example, we can see cognitivist principles where the child is consciously developing a style of handwriting. The act of writing is taking up much less of their concentration so they are now in a position to refine their skill. If our example contained more detail about the learner's personality and their response to different activities, we would undoubtedly see more cognitivist principles at work.

Cognitivist design principles and activities include the following:

- Pre-tests check whether the correct network of knowledge is present before trying to add to it. Feedback from pre-tests links to material to fill in any gaps uncovered. Pre-tests are also intended to activate the existing network of knowledge making the process of assimilation or accommodation easier for the learner.

- Advance organisers are used at the beginning of new topics to sum up what learners have covered so far. This, again, is intended to reactivate their existing knowledge network.

- Points or topics in the learning material are broken into between five and nine distinct sections to make optimum use of short-term memory.

- A visual map of the network of topics and sections in the resource is provided. This representation is intended to help the learner form mental connections between topics and see how they converge to form a body of knowledge or complete skill. Menu systems can be used to illustrate this effectively.

- Functional and visual continuity should be kept throughout the resource. This means the menu, content and buttons are shown in the same place and have the same appearance from page to page. Changes in visual continuity should only be used to draw attention to specific points or functional changes (i.e. using bold type to draw attention to points or making the 'submit' button in an assessment visibly distinct from other buttons).
- Opportunities should be provided to apply the new knowledge in parallel with existing knowledge. The intention is that if the learner has to synthesise the new information to apply it to a familiar problem (the existing knowledge) then deeper learning and therefore better assimilation or accommodation will occur.
- Materials, activities and support structures are provided in a variety of media and formats to cater for differences in learning style.

Constructivist theory

Constructivist theory bears more than a passing resemblance to cognitivist theory. It states that knowledge is constructed in the mind of the learner through perception of experiences. This underlines something that all schools of learning advocate: that learning is achieved through activity. Constructivist theory is different in that it recognises that different lessons can be learned from the same experience, depending on how each individual perceives it. It also states that learning is contextual and that learners may apply the same principles in different ways depending on the situation they are in. This implies that the authenticity of learning activities plays a part in the lessons learned.

The constructivist school is divided over one point: the role of social interaction in this process. Some such as Piaget [14] believe that social interaction plays an important part in learning. Others (the social constructivists including Vygotsky [15]) believe that learning is not just an activity, it is a social activity. If you consider that feedback comes from another human being (whether delivered by a computer program or in other interactions) then this can be seen as true. However, this viewpoint is often interpreted in social constructivist design as 'nothing is learned without long debate among peers'. Adopting this strategy along with the common practice of linking interaction into the assessment criteria can create a situation where those who are field independent are forced to take part in activities before they are in a position to benefit from them [16]. This can lead to disengagement and limited learning as a result.

Our example shows constructivist theory at work in their schooldays and beyond.

This approach sees the role of the teacher as providing relevant experiences and providing supporting social activities aimed at guiding interpretation of those experiences. This is a very similar model to the cognitivist one, but the emphasis is usually on the individual's learning being created in a process of negotiation between peers and the tutor.

Constructivist design principles and activities include:

- problem solving in case-based scenarios;
- group work, usually on case-based problems;
- role play;
- forum posting with comments on peer postings;
- forum submissions being part of the assessment strategy;
- points for reflective exercises;
- the tutor as 'guide on the side' as opposed to 'sage on the stage'.

Connectivist and situated perspectives

The situated perspective [17] recognises that learning happens in a social or cultural context and the context plays a central role in the knowledge construction of a learner. Situationism can be seen as considering knowledge to be a part of a culture. For example, the skills, attitudes, behaviours and knowledge that combine to form what many would see as a good doctor are created and maintained by the community of practising doctors. Institutions may add formality to the definition of a good doctor, but those institutions are usually made up of senior and respected members of the community of practice. Another aspect of the situationist perspective is that learners start at the edges of the community. At first they have limited interaction with those at the centre of the community but learn what is expected of them if they are to be an accepted member of that community. It is as if the learner sets their own objectives based on the knowledge, skills and behaviours valued by the culture in the community of practice they belong to.

When the learner starts displaying some of the skills, behaviours, attitudes and knowledge they are expected to acquire (possibly from your resource), they start playing a more active role in the community of practice. Over time, they learn more and take up a more central role; they start mentoring and teaching others, eventually playing a part in determining the cultural view of how a good doctor should behave and practise.

This perspective on learning would consider the teacher and the learner as the same person playing different roles in their community. The implication for learning is that the culture plays a large part in setting the curriculum and the learner sets their objectives to align with this.

The connectivist perspective

Connectivism is an emerging perspective that has similarities to situationism. It considers the learner to be part of a whole. The perspectives differ in that connectivism sees that whole as a network rather than a culture. It also considers learning to be 'the process of building networks of information, contacts and resources that are applied to real problems' [18]. The emphasis for connectivism is on knowing how and where to find relevant, good-quality information to tackle the problem at hand.

It does not advocate adding that information to a cognitive schema within the learner and considers the external network of information as a cognitive schema in its own right. It can be seen as considering learning to be within a network that the individual accesses and contributes to as opposed to being within the learner themselves.

In a world where core information and evidence is changing rapidly, learning and maintaining a complete body of knowledge appears to be an increasingly unrealistic goal. Designing courses that address this issue formally will be one of the main challenges for the future of e-learning and is where perspectives like these may prove to be invaluable.

Situationist and connectivist activities could include:

- masterclasses and tutorials;
- blogging and reading professional or alumni blogs;
- use of portfolios, especially when made public;
- publication of research and other peer review activities;
- teaching and mentoring;
- informal learning experiences like conference workshops;
- learners setting their own objectives;
- work generated during a course becoming part of its learning materials.

Ally [3] sums up the three main theories by saying that 'behaviourist strategies can be used to teach the facts (what), cognitivist strategies the principles and processes (how), and constructivist strategies the real-life and personal applications and contextual learning'. The situationist and connectivist perspectives are a movement toward formalising commonly used informal learning strategies and go some way to providing us with an insight into the roles that society and technology can play when learners begin to take ownership of their development. They also provide design principles and activities that are appropriate for learners at the later stages of their professional development or those approaching mastery of a discipline.

4.2.3 Learning in the digital age

With the development and proliferation of e-learning in all its formats, there has been a focus on learning in and for the digital age. Prenksy [19] describes digital natives, the so-called y or x generation and digital immigrants, and what might essentially be described as a paradigm shift required to engage and educate 'modern' learners. In the last decades of the 20th century, he argues that young people have grown up immersed in a digital world – he describes them as digital natives. The learning and teaching expectations of digital natives are totally different from those of other, older generations. Prensky describes the situation:

> Today's students have not just changed incrementally from those of the past . . . A really big discontinuity has taken place . . . the arrival and rapid dissemination of digital technology in the last decades of the 20th century.

Where does this leave the rest of us? Again Prensky describes the concept of the 'digital immigrant' – someone who has adopted technology at a later stage in their life. Typically, of course, the digital immigrant will be the educator and the digital native is the student, and Prensky proposes that there is a significant disconnect between teaching methods and the learning requirements. Digital immigrants:

> who themselves learned – and so choose to teach – slowly, step-by-step, one thing at a time, individually, and above all, seriously.

Digital natives:

> are used to receiving information really fast. They like to parallel-process and multi-task. They prefer their graphics before their text rather than the opposite. They prefer random access (like hypertext). They function best when networked. They thrive on instant gratification and frequent rewards. They prefer games to 'serious' work.

So it appears that the huge challenge to educators is to change delivery methods and content to suit those who learn in different ways from the traditional 'tried and tested' model. Prensky argues that: 'Today's teachers have to learn to communicate in the language and style of their students.' and '"Future" content is to a large extent, not surprisingly, digital and technological.'

4.3 The course

We will describe the elements of the course structure under the headings of:
- navigation;
- page/screen structure;
- materials/activities;

- assessments;
- choosing a platform.

The course structure is the point where your materials, activities and support systems come together to form an online environment for learning. We will touch on cognitivist principles and others to design or evaluate an effective scaffolding for learning [3]. This scaffolding aims to do the following:

- Create an intuitive structure. If the resource is not clearly structured then the trainee spends more time learning how to get around and less time on the material.
- Facilitate accommodation and assimilation [3].
- Map the material.
- Rejuvenate or expand learner motivations.

4.3.1 Navigation

The navigation provides a map. This map provides your learners with an overview of the area you will be teaching and can help them understand the relationship between the topics and points you will be addressing. The method of navigation you choose and how it is structured are key to generating a good map of your teaching.

It is important to keep your navigation in the same place and to have the same structure on every page. Maintaining the same structure builds in resolved redundancy [3] and maintaining the same location for it allows the learner to focus on the materials rather than the structure they are in.

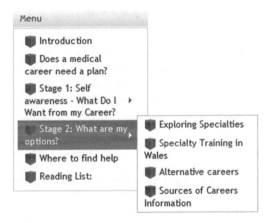

Figure 4.3 Teaching map

4.3.2 Page or screen structure

There are a number of features that should be present on the first page. These are as follows:

- Show what will be expected of the learner. This includes their expected time commitment and information about any final work to be submitted.
- Provide an outline of what technology they will need to be able to take part fully in the course. This could be as simple as stating they will need the latest version of a web browser and access to a word-processing package.
- Clearly signpost where the learner can access the support structures you have in place. Ideally there will be a 'support' item in the main navigation.

Be aware that they may only read the information on the first page once. The next time they visit they will hopefully use the navigation to pick up directly from where they left off. The other pages in your resource should follow cognitivist design principles to make sure that there is little distraction from the message you are trying to convey or the activity you are asking them to take part in. The first page in each topic should provide an overview of what the learner previously covered and how the resource relates to the rest of the training programme. This is your first opportunity to bolster your learners' motivations [2] by outlining the personal and professional benefits of taking part. Advanced organisers should be included at the start of each topic. These outline what the learner has covered and how it relates to the coming material. This also provides another opportunity to rejuvenate flagging motivations.

4.3.3 Course materials and activities

You will need to start building your resource by gathering learning materials to cover the topics and points in the course structure you wrote. Once you have the materials (or a good idea of what they will be), you can look at adding activities to your resource.

To add appropriate activities, you will need to take another look at the objectives and determine what activity would be likely to demonstrate them. The way to determine the best activity is to look at the verb in the objective and choose a theory of learning that is likely to meet it (behaviourist for facts; cognitivist strategies to demonstrate principles and processes at work; constructivist strategies to demonstrate real-life and personal applications and contextual learning). Once you consider the design principles and activities for each, you should be able to determine the best activity. The next step is to consider the course structure and determine at which point the learner is likely to be able to demonstrate the objective. This is where you add your activity.

These activities are the basis of your resource and will probably play a major role in your assessment strategy. There will also be points when you can see that other activities need to be added for the learner to progress from one topic or point to another. Again, keep in mind the various learning theories; these will help guide your decisions.

There is a practical point you need to consider before moving on. The activities may include forums, wikis or other technologies. If they do, you need to make sure the learner has experience of using these technologies before applying them to their learning. You can make sure of this by adding plenary activities aimed at providing:

- the opportunity to rehearse the technologies they will be using further on;
- an opportunity to investigate the course structure (especially the support structures);
- an opportunity to find out about their peers (if this is a feature of the course).

Use your learner profiles to determine what task is suitable for the plenary sessions and, if possible, place them close enough to the learning activities so that learners still remember how to use the technologies you introduced.

4.4 The assessment

Assessment is a specialist subject in its own right and deserves far more attention than we can give it within this chapter. One key aspect of assessment is that it is inextricably linked with the learning objectives for the education piece; assessment must map to the learning objectives. The reason for this is clear – learners do not expect to be assessed on subject matter that has not been signposted to them in the learning objectives and conversely if, as a teacher, you do not set learning objectives, you will not know what to teach and your audience will not know what they are supposed to learn; also you will not know what to assess. If your learning pieces do not include some form of assessment, your audience will not be able to determine what they have learned. So how do we write good learning objectives? There are some clear guidelines [20] on this which link in with Bloom's taxonomy of learning, as previously explained.

4.4.1 Writing learning objectives (further examples) [21]

Learning objectives are essentially statements of what learners should be able to do if they have acquired knowledge and skills from the learning piece. A typical learning objective takes the following form.

- *Stem*: at the end of this (session, course, topic, etc.) the learner should be able to. . . .
- *List of tasks*: demonstrating mastery of what has been learned. The task statements will contain verbs such as show, calculate, decide, list, explain, apply, estimate, derive, design, choose, critique etc. NOTE: The verbs used must be measurable or observable, so words like understand, know, appreciate etc. are inappropriate here.
- *Definition of the task*: a statement of what is required.
- *Optionally* a statement of the conditions under which the task is to be carried out.

Here are two examples:

- At the end of this session, the learner will be able to list four key components of adult-learning theory.
- At the end of this session, the learner will be able to, under examination conditions, perform a theoretical calculation of the partial pressure of oxygen in the blood from a set of relevant data presented, explaining why a theoretical calculation might differ from an empirical situation involving a real patient.

4.4.2 Evidence of completion

With larger e-learning or blended learning projects, there is often the need to provide evidence of learner completion and other metrics showing learner uptake, improvement of incident rates, or compliance with institutional objectives even before the first cohort has graduated.

This is the case because there is a fundamental difference between education and training. One way to consider the difference is to look at the focus of outcomes. The outcome of education focuses primarily on the development of the individual, whereas the primary focus of training is on the development of the institution or industry. If a training programme does not offer professional development of workers and some way to demonstrate improvement then it will get limited support. It is also true that if training programmes offer limited opportunities for personal development, they will get limited support from learners.

4.5 Choosing a platform

A platform is the means of delivering your message to your learners. Each platform has its own characteristics and features.

We can roughly divide electronic platforms into two categories, each containing a variety of media types. These are *connected* and *disconnected* platforms. The defining characteristic of connected media is that the platform presents information held in an external location, so a change to the external source changes the information the learner receives. This allows information to be updated and distributed quickly. Connected platforms can be defined for our purposes as 'information fed to the client machine via a network platform'.

Disconnected media are the other end of the spectrum. The information is held within the platform and cannot be updated. We can define it as 'information hard-wired into its platform'. DVDs, CD-ROMs and PDFs are all examples of disconnected platforms. You may access the PDF online but the information in the PDF is permanent. Changing it would mean creating a new file.

Be aware of what reports will be expected and choose the systems that are capable of delivering this information as painlessly as possible. You may need to generate regular reports detailing course activity well before the first cohort has graduated.

4.6 Summary

The key to using e-teaching is to prepare. This preparation takes into account the needs of all of the stakeholders, but with the focus on the learners. Plan the design of the resource in a systemic way, utilising a project scope approach. Build in evaluation and QA from the beginning. When at the point of constructing the resources, revisit learning outcomes that will drive the content, activities and assessments. Take care about navigation and be wary of overloading each page on the screen with too much distraction.

References

1 Waller KV. Writing Instructional Objectives. The National Accrediting Agency for Clinical Laboratory Sciences (NAACLS). [Online] 2010. [Cited: 7 February 2011]. http://www.naacls.org/docs/announcement/writing-objectives.pdf.

2 ODL QC. Buyers Guide: The Course. ODL QC – The Open and Distance Learning Quality Council – Buyers Guide to Distance Learning. [Online] [Cited: 17 March 2011]. http://www.odlqc.org.uk/buyers2.htm.

3 Ally M. Foundations of Educational Theory for Online Learning. [book auth.] Terry Anderson and Fathi Elloumi. Theory and Practice of Online Learning. Athabasca: Athabasca University, 2004:3–26.

4 Mayer RE. Multimedia Learning. Cambridge University Press, New York, 2005.

5 Krathwohl DR. A Revision of Bloom's Taxonomy: An Overview. [Online] Ohio State University, Autumn 2002. [Cited: 24 February 2011]. http://www.unco.edu/cetl/sir/stating_outcome/documents/Krathwohl.pdf.

6 Simpson O. Supporting Students in Online, Open and Distance Learning. Second edition. RoutlegeFalmer, Oxon, 2002.

7   Google. Google Analytics | Official website. Google Analytics. [Online] [Cited: 12 August 2011]. http://www.google.com/intl/en/analytics/.

8   Aubry M. Piwik, Open source tracking. Piwik. [Online] OpenX. [Cited: 12 August 2011]. http://piwik.org/.

9   Butterfield S, Chambers M, Mosely B, Prebble T, Uys P, Woodhouse D. External Quality Assurance for the Virtual Insitution. New Zealand Universities Academic Audit Unit, Wellingon, 1999, AAU Series on Quality;4. ISSN:11748826.

10   Kuomi J. Quality is better ensured by practitioners than by researchers. In: D Sewart (ed.), One World Many Voices: quality in open and distance learning. Birmingham: s.n., 1995. selected papers from the 17th World Conference of International Council for Distance Education.

11   Bereiter C, Scardamalia M. Rethinking learning: Handbook of education and human development: New models of learning, teaching and schooling. Blackwell, Cambridge, MA, 1996:485–513.

12   Ally M. Theory and Practice of Online Learning. Second edition. Terry Anderson (ed.). AU Press, Athabasca, 2008.

13   Ormrod JE. Human learning. Third edition. Prentice-Hall, Upper Saddle River, NJ, 1999.

14   Summary of Jean Piaget's life and theories, Wikipedia.org. [Cited 19 January 2012]. http://en.wikipedia.org/wiki/Jean_Piaget.

15   Summary of Lev Vygotsky's life and theories, Wikipedia.org. [Cited 19 January 2012] http://en.wikipedia.org/wiki/Vygotsky.

16   Witkin HA, Moore CA, Goodenough DR, Cox PW. Field-dependent and field-independent cognitive styles and their educational implications. American Educational Research Association, Review of Educational Research 1977;47:1–64.

17   Brown J, Collins A, Duguid P. Situated cognition and the culture of learning. Educational Researcher 1989;18:32–42.

18   Anderson T, Dron J. Three Generations of Distance Education Pedagogy. The International Review of Research in Open and Distance Learning March 2011;12(3).

19   Prensky M. On the Horizon: MCB University Press October 2001;9(5). http://www.marcprensky.com/writing/Prensky%20-%20Digital%20Natives,%20Digital%20Immigrants%20-%20Part1.pdf.

20   Anderson WL, Krathwohl D. A Taxonomy for Learning, Teaching, and Assessing: A Revision of Bloom's Taxonomy of Educational Objectives, Abridged Edition. Allyn & Bacon, 2000. ISBN: 080131903X.

21   Felder RM, Brent R. The ABCs of Engineering Education: ABET, Bloom's taxonomy, cooperative learning, and so on. North Carolina State University/ Education Designs Inc. American Society for Engineering Education, 2004. [Cited 14 October 2011]. http://scholar.googleusercontent.com/scholar?q=cache:Adks4GgBdqsJ:scholar.google.com/+THE+ABC%E2%80%99S+OF+ENGINEERING+EDUCATION:&hl=en&as_sdt=1,5.

Chapter 5 **Access to e-learning**

In this chapter we will be looking at a range of e-learning systems and media. We will consider each from the point of view of someone who is planning on using them to learn. For those intending to use the systems described as part of a course, this chapter will provide some insight into how learners can use these systems to best effect and help you to design your course structures and activities accordingly.

A range of plugins and other peripherals will be mentioned throughout this chapter. These can make the transition from traditional to online learning much easier, but technology changes at such a rate that any examples mentioned by name will probably have been superseded by something else soon after publication. For this reason, we would encourage you to take a look at any examples provided but also to make your own investigations to see what is available.

5.1 The basics: files and folders

There are only so many times you can think 'where is that paper I read on . . . ' and then spend the best part of an afternoon trying to find a specific citation. Sooner or later you find that e-learning will only be an efficient use of time if it is approached in an efficient way. Since arriving at this conclusion, we tested a number of filing systems to find the most intuitive and efficient system. We share our findings with you in the hope that these basic measures save you hours of frustration.

First, create a folder purely for your learning. In this folder, create another folder for the year. Inside the year folder, create a new folder for the course you are on now. In this folder you must try to resist the urge to create folders

How to Succeed at E-learning, First Edition. Peter Donnelly, Joel Benson, and Paul Kirk.
© 2012 John Wiley & Sons Ltd. Published 2012 by John Wiley & Sons Ltd.

for each of the assignments and throw everything to do with that assignment into the folder. It is easier to find materials later if you create folders that mirror the course structure (including the assignments) and save any downloads or work to folders named after the topic they are associated with.

If you have material from previous courses, move it over to this file structure so all your learning is in the same file system. You will be referring to previous courses and their materials throughout your career, so having them in the same filing system will make finding previous material much easier.

Having this file and folder system on one computer is very useful but risky. If the computer breaks or is lost, so is the coursework. If we make a portable version on a USB flash drive, we can access our coursework from virtually any computer. The problem we have with this system is that if we work on the flash drive and a number of other computers, it can be tricky to synchronise the multiple versions. Another alternative is to use an online system for your files. This way you will have a single version on multiple computers or devices simultaneously and will have no problem synchronising or accessing your work.

SkyDrive [1], Dropbox [2] and iCloud [3] are examples of cloud or online file storage systems. You create an account with the company (usually via their downloadable software or website) and can upload files and folders to a location online. At the time of writing, at least one company provides a limited amount of storage and an account at no cost. Some also provide software to allow the files and folders to appear on your computer in the same way as all the other files and folders do. Some also provide software for other devices, allowing you to access your coursework and research from supported mobile devices. These systems can also offer other features like:

- the ability to recover previous versions and deleted files;
- the option of sharing files with other people.

These systems reduce the risk of losing work and help manage versions. Another huge advantage of using a system like this is that you can use the spare 10 minutes in your day to carry on with your learning via any supported mobile device with access to the Internet.

Whether you choose one of the suggestions here or decide on another, the main concern is that your work is safe and that you can find the latest version of it quickly.

5.2 Security

The vast majority of threats to your computer are spread via the Internet and email. If you do not protect yourself from these threats, it is likely that your computer will become infected very quickly. The effects of infection can result in your computer being so slow or cluttered with pop-up windows that it is rendered useless. In the worst case scenarios, it can result in the theft of your work or identity. Either way, infection will seriously disrupt your study plans.

Once you are infected, it can be very difficult to put your computer right so prevention with a good suite of security tools is essential for anyone who intends to learn or research online. A key issue is to ensure that you update regularly.

5.3 The book and the browser

Before we look at web pages, it is worth considering how we use books. I have two types of book. The first is for entertainment and this usually contains a simple marker or the occasional turned corner. The other type is reference books; these are well thumbed, have pencilled or highlighted notes in the margins and sticky notes protruding from the top. This is because these books show the evidence of the strategies used to make them serve learning needs more efficiently.

Although the modern website is far more interactive than paper, we can employ the same strategies we use for learning from books when learning from websites. To convert our strategies from books to websites, we will need to have sticky notes and the ability to scribble directly on the pages. We will also need to be able to take a searchable copy of the pages in which we are interested.

Taking searchable copies is important for two reasons. The first is so we can overcome one major difference between books and websites; the fact that your web page may have changed or disappeared the next time you visit. The second reason is to take advantage of another major difference between web pages and paper; the fact that digital media is searchable. If web pages are saved in a format that is searchable, it becomes possible to search for a citation not just in one document but in every document on your computer. This strategy can enable you to find the citation you need in seconds as opposed to hours. It also regularly provides useful results from sources you may not have considered looking through.

In an ideal world, all the features I have mentioned would be available in a single browser that is purpose-built for research and education. Unfortunately this browser has not been invented yet, but thankfully the flexibility built into some of the most popular web browsers available today can provide us with the features we need.

5.3.1 Browsers
There is a wide variety of web browsers available, but the most popular are Firefox [4], Opera [5], Chrome [6], Safari [7] and Internet Explorer [8].

There are two areas where all browsers differ; the first is in how they display web pages. Complex web applications like VLEs may not function properly in one browser, but may work well in another. The other major difference is that each one has a different set of features and a different range of add-ons we can use to support our learning and teaching more effectively.

Firefox has the widest range of add-ons at this time, but you will need at least one other browser to be sure you can access every feature on every website. The second most reliable browser is likely to be the one that comes with your computer by default. For Windows users, this would be Internet Explorer; Apple Mac users would have Safari.

Once you have chosen and installed a browser for your learning, you will need to add the features that will help you apply your offline learning strategies to the online world.

5.3.2 Bookmarks

All modern web browsers have systems for collecting bookmarks. Bookmarks can be organised in a folder structure that closely resembles the structure you use to organise your coursework. Figure 5.1 shows how a bookmark toolbar can be used effectively to organise daily browsing and your learning or research. This example is my bookmark strategy for writing this and other chapters in this book.

The last three items are the most important for online learning. 'Libraries' contains links to Google Scholar [9] and PUBMED [10]. Other useful sites are available including BioMed Central [11] the TRIP database [12] and Medscape [13]. If you are already on a course or part of an academic institution, it is also worth adding their library to this folder. The bookmarks you add to this folder are aimed at providing a starting point for any online research you do.

The 'Courses' bookmark contains three folders. We suggest the following system for organising your course bookmarks. The first folder is called 'Past' and holds all the bookmarks for past courses. The second is the 'Future' and contains a selection of courses you aim to do one day.

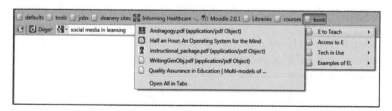

Figure 5.1 Example of effective bookmarking

The third item is the course or project you are working on now. It is wise to give this its own folder to stop the inevitable amount of clutter from getting in the way of your current project. Once a course, module or project is completed, it can be dragged from the toolbar into the appropriate part of the 'Past' folder. This helps retain useful bookmarks while keeping your bookmarks toolbar clear enough to work with.

There are also a number of alternative approaches to bookmarking that show great promise. These involve saving copies of bookmarked pages in a website. You can then log in to the website to organise your bookmarks. Some companies also offer browser add-ons and plugins for viewing directly from your browser. The advantage of systems like these is that your bookmark collection is available to you from more than one browser and is not lost if your computer breaks down. These approaches also offer a number of other possibilities including the ability to share certain parts of your collection with others and to see what bookmarks they may be sharing. Some of the current offerings are Delicious [14], Google Bookmarks (part of Google Apps) [15], Zoho [16], Diigo [17] and Webnotes [18]. Many of these can provide an all-in-one solution to your online teaching or learning needs and are well worth trying out. The authors have extensively tested one of these offerings called Diigo. It has a range of very useful features that are focused on use in an educational context. It also offers the opportunity to join collaborative communities and share in their findings.

5.3.3 Retaining copies of your pages

It has already been said that taking searchable copies of web pages is one way to make sure you can guarantee access to pages in the future. Some websites provide material in PDFs and these can be directly saved to your computer. If the page you want is not a format that is easy to save, there are still many options available for taking hard copies. Just be sure that your chosen method is searchable. If it is not, you may struggle to find the citation you need from your ever-growing collection of sources.

Converting your most valuable web pages to PDFs is a good way to prevent valuable sources from disappearing, but some PDF makers are not capable of recognising text. They just take a snapshot image of the page and do not index the text so that you can search through it at a later date. Adobe Acrobat [19] is about the most comprehensive PDF tool available at the time of writing, but freeware PDF generators like 7-PDF [20] are available that do recognise text.

One advantage of good PDF documents is that they can be searched in a very flexible way. Adobe Acrobat Reader [21] has the option to search for text in one PDF, but also provides the option to search through an entire collection of PDFs.

5.3.4 Sticky notes and annotations

One of the strategies you can use with traditional books is to highlight the passage that interests you on a bookmarked page. Without this, you can find yourself at a loss to remember why you added the bookmark in the first place. There are tools available for writing directly on a web page so that you can easily trace the part you are interested in. It is also possible to add a sticky note in a corner that you can add further comments to. This is invaluable in tracing your thoughts at a later date. There are stand-alone plugins for browsers to add these features, but we suggest it is better to use a solution that incorporates your bookmarks with your other research and collaboration tools. Diigo [17], Zoho [16] and Webnotes [18] are some providers that offer this functionality.

5.4 Collaborative research

Collaboration is often an essential part of teaching and learning in online medical education and we will take a closer look at how to get the most from these experiences soon. For now, we will address the fact that the Internet is not just a library. It is also a place where groups of like-minded individuals can share experience, best practice and resources. Linking in with these groups can provide good-quality solutions to a whole range of problems and also give you access to a global perspective on many topics.

Some of the research and collaboration tools already mentioned provide access to groups and other collaboration tools. A quick search of one of these tools [17] for 'medical education' revealed 215 groups with memberships ranging from zero to over 200. Some of the higher-quality medical and medical education forums on the Internet include New Media Medicine [22], Student Doc [23] and Doctors.net.uk [24].

5.4.1 Making best use of forums and wikis

Whether you are learning or teaching with forums and wikis, it is important to recognise that they are not simply an online version of the classroom. A classroom offers the opportunity to get an immediate response to a question. This immediacy is very helpful in revealing underlying assumptions or prejudices that can then be addressed. If we are addressing these in-classroom group activities, the group process of forming, storming, norming, and performing [25] can happen far more rapidly because it is happening without the mediation of technology.

Forums and wikis may not offer unmediated immediacy but they do offer something else. The mediation involved with posting and waiting for replies provides the chance to give a considered standpoint. If the activity and topic play to this strength, forums can provide very rich learning experiences.

Getting to grips with forum and wiki tools can take some time. Add to this the fact that the rest of the course environment may be new to you and it is easy to see that if you do not take full advantage of any plenary sessions offered, you may find yourself lagging behind when the course starts in earnest. Take the time to introduce yourself and practise using the forums. This is just as true for new tutors as it is for learners. The following points are based on what alumni from various e-learning courses wished they had done when first starting their courses:

1 *Get into the forums early and practise*: we reiterate this because we cannot stress how important this point is. Make sure you find out how the quote tool works; it will be invaluable if you are asked to comment on your peers' posts later in the course.

2 *Use a text editor or word processor for your replies*: it is not uncommon for learners or tutors to spend time carefully crafting a reply to a post. When they click 'submit', they find that their web browser asks for their login again and the post they wrote has been lost. The solution to this is to write your reply in a text editor of some sort. Once you are happy with your reply, you can copy and paste it into the forum window and click 'submit'. If you are then asked for your login, you can cut and paste your carefully crafted reply back into the forum and your time has not been wasted.

3 *Use the appropriate netiquette*: there are usually rules for how and what to post to a forum. These rules are designed to make sure everyone is treated with respect and provided with the richest educational environment possible. Most of the time you will find the rules in the FAQ section of the forum, which is usually accessible from the home page. These rules usually include variations on the following:

  • *Be professional:* on public forums it is not uncommon to find that someone has posted something deliberately inflammatory or just completely pointless. It has also been known to happen on institutional forums. While their post may dismiss everything you believe, resist the urge to post your opinion straight back. Type your response into a text document and ask yourself three questions. The first is 'Would I say this to their face?' The next question is 'Would I be happy to see this published with my name against it?' Don't forget that once something is online, the whole world may be able to see it. The final question is 'Would this add something constructive to the topic in this thread?' If the answer to any of these questions is no, it may be best to either rewrite your post or report the abuse to the forum moderator privately.

- *Be kind*: someone much like you will be reading the post. Ask how you would feel if you received it. It is also wise to assume that if someone has made an offensive post, the offence was unintentional. Ask whoever sent the post to clarify their point before you respond.

- *Be yourself*: your personality is a vital part of any point you make; it is your view of this world and is an important part of your posts. At first it is very difficult to follow these rules and still be yourself. Over time you will find that you become more comfortable with using forums and find that your posts will convey your points and personality quite clearly. At this point you may start to feel like you have joined a community rather than just added to a web page.

- *Be clear and concise*: keeping up with a busy forum can be very time-consuming. Try to make your point in as short a post as possible. If you have more than one point to make, maybe you could use one post for each point. Also, read each post through before you click 'submit' and ask yourself if it could be taken in unintended ways. If so, rewrite it before submitting. Doing this can take up extra time initially, but it may end up saving considerable time and embarrassment from explaining that you did not mean the post quite in the way it was taken. If someone gets offended, it can take considerable effort to rebuild your working relationship with them.

- *Be considerate with formatting*: the formatting, colours and fonts you use can make a difference to how easy it is to read your posts. Use capitals sparingly. In forums, using capitals is considered SHOUTING. It also can make your post more difficult to read. Keep your paragraphs as short as possible to make it easier for members to read and find the part they would like to quote.

- *Be on-topic*: everyone struggles to find the time to keep up with a busy forum. Reading through a thread that suddenly digresses into what is happening in the news disrupts the flow of the forum and makes it difficult for people to keep track of the topic discussion. If you do want to pick up on something that is off-topic, you can usually send a private message to the other member. It is equally disruptive to post a question or response in the wrong forum. Most people new to forums do this at least once. If you cannot remove the post, it is worth replying to it with a short apology. If your tutor cannot see your post in the correct forum, there is also a chance you may lose out on assessment marks. Consistently cross-posting is considered to be spam. If you do this, you may find members start adding you to their 'blocked' list.

- *Post early*: forum activities usually have a limited time span. If you post the day before the activity is over, you will have very few responses. You will get insight from other people's posts but without responses to your own, you will find that your understanding of the topic has gone unchallenged and may not have grown as much as it could have. Posting late will also mean that your group will not benefit from any insight you may have.

- *Set times for posting*: consider the forum activities as 'going to classes' and allocate shorter but very regular times to visit. You will find it much easier to keep up with the discussion and will also be able to see how much is being posted. This will help you decide whether you need to set aside more time to keep up with that particular topic.

These tips will help with forums and are equally valid for wikis, but some online activities may require you to work in a group with more structure. These structured groups usually have a leader or editor and are common in wiki activities. The group will commonly allocate tasks to its members and work together to create an end-product. Allocating roles and tasks and deciding what goes into the end-product takes more time than it would in a classroom situation. The next section looks at some of the options available for making the most of these types of group.

5.4.2 Using software to manage group work effectively

During an online course, it is likely that you will be asked to take part in group work with peers. The first stage usually involves you being allocated to a group and given a role. Sometimes the tutor may allow you to decide on the group you wish to join and let the group decide on the roles each member will take.

At this point, your group will need to discuss the activity that has been assigned and share ideas on how it can be tackled. This process is called 'forming' [22] and can take valuable time to be resolved. One way you can speed up this process and get to know your group a little better is by arranging a conference call for your group using software like Skype [26], GoToMeeting [27] or SightSpeed [28]. These allow you to video- or voice-call more than one person simultaneously. Most of them provide a number of features that will allow you to share links and desktop applications, and take notes of what was decided at the meeting. They do require you to have speakers, a microphone or webcam but most modern laptops and mobile phones have these features built into them as standard.

If you can use conference or video calling, the first item your group should discuss (after introductions) is who is going to take notes. This is important supporting documentation for your group project and will be vital for showing who has made what contributions. Without this, it will be extremely difficult for your tutor to allocate assessment marks fairly.

Your conference call may go so well that your group decides it would like to continue the activity using the conference software rather than the software provided by the tutor. This is something you must discuss with your tutor before proceeding. The reason for this is that even though Skype and others may provide more features and a more intuitive interface for group working, most educational group activity software has reporting, tracking and feedback tools that provide tutors with the information they need to assess contributions accurately. Without this information, the tutor and individuals in your group will be at a disadvantage.

References

1 Microsoft. Windows Live SkyDrive – Online document storage and file sharing. Windows Live. [Online] Microsoft, 2011. [Cited: 18 September 2011]. http://explore.live.com/skydrive.

2 Dropbox. Dropbox – Features – Simplify your life. [Online] Dropbox, 2011. [Cited: 18 September 2011]. http://www.dropbox.com/features.

3 Apple Inc. Apple – iCloud stores your content and pushes it directly to all your devices. Apple. [Online] Apple Inc, 2011. [Cited: 18 September 2011]. http://www.apple.com/icloud/what-is.html.

4 Mozilla Firefox. Mozilla Firefox Web Browser. [Online] Mozilla Project. [Cited: 28 May 2011]. http://www.mozilla.com/en-US/firefox/fx/.

5 Opera Software. Opera Products. Opera Browser | Faster and safer Internet | free download. [Online] Opera Software. [Cited: 28 May 2011]. http://www.opera.com/products/.

6 Google. Google Chrome – The Web is what you make of it. [Online] Google. [Cited: 28 May 2011]. http://www.google.com/chrome/intl/en/make/download.html?brand=CHKZ.

7 Apple. Apple Safari – Browse the web in more powerful ways. Apple. [Online] Apple. [Cited: 28 May 2011]. http://www.apple.com/safari/.

8 Microsoft. Internet Explorer – Microsoft Windows. Windows. [Online] Microsoft. [Cited: 28 May 2011]. http://windows.microsoft.com/en-US/internet-explorer/products/ie/home.

9 Google. Google Scholar. Google Scholar. [Online] [Cited: 18 May 2011]. http://scholar.google.co.uk/.

10 PUBMED. [Online] [Cited: 18 May 2011]. http://www.ncbi.nlm.nih.gov/pubmed.

11   Springer Science+Business Media. BioMed Central – The Open Access Publisher. BioMed Central. [Online] Springer Science+Business Media. [Cited: 12 June 2011]. http://www.biomedcentral.com/.

12   TRIP Database Limited. Trip Database – clinical search engine. TRIP Database. [Online] TRIP Database Limited. [Cited: 9 June 2011]. http://www.tripdatabase.com/.

13   WebMD Health Professional Network. Medscape home page. Medscape. [Online] WebMD. [Cited: 9 June 2011]. http://www.medscape.com/.

14   Yahoo. Delicious. [Online] Yahoo. [Cited: 9 June 2011]. http://www.delicious.com/.

15   Google. Google Bookmarks. Google Docs. [Online] Gooogle. [Cited: 9 June 2011]. https://www.google.com/bookmarks.

16   Zohocorp. Zoho Home page. Zoho. [Online] Zohocorp. [Cited: 9 June 2011]. https://www.zoho.com/.

17   Diigo . Diigo Home page. Diigo.com. [Online] Diigo. [Cited: 9 June 2011]. http://www.diigo.com/index.

18   Webnotes.inc. Webnotes Home page. Webnotes.com. [Online] [Cited: 9 June 2011]. http://www.webnotes.net/.

19   Adobe. Adobe Acrobat X Pro. Adobe Acrobat X Pro. [Online] Adobe inc. [Cited: 9 June 2011]. http://acrobat.buy.uk.sem.adobe.com/content/a10_pro?sdid=IBNCB&skwcid=TC|22705|adobe%20acrobat%20x||S|e|8383552024.

20   7-PDF. 7-PFD home page. 7-PDF. [Online] 7-PDF. [Cited: 9 June 2011]. http://www.7-pdf.de/.

21   Adobe. Adobe Reader X. Adobe Reader X. [Online] [Cited: 9 June 2011]. http://www.adobe.com/uk/products/reader.html.

22   New Media Medicine. New Media | Medicine. New Media Medicine. [Online] New Media Medicine Ltd. [Cited: 12 June 2011]. http://www.newmediamedicine.com/forum/content/137-about-new-media-medicine.html.

23   Student Doc. Medical School Forum. Student Doc. [Online] Student Doc. [Cited: 12 June 2011]. http://www.studentdoc.com/phpBB2/.

24   Doctors.net.uk. Doctors.net.uk – Forum. Doctors.net.uk. [Online] Doctors.net.uk. [Cited: 12 June 2011]. http://about.doctors.net.uk/Member-Benefits/Forum.

25   Tuckman BW. Developmental Sequence in Small Groups. Psychological Bulletin 1965;63(6):384–399.

26   Skype Limited. Conference calls – Video conferencing. Skype. [Online] Skype Limited, 2011. [Cited: 25 July 2011]. http://www.skype.com/intl/en/home.

27   Citrix Online, UK Ltd. Web Conferencing | GoToMeeting. GoToMeeting. [Online] Citrix Online, UK Ltd, 2011. [Cited: 25 July 2011]. http://www.gotomeeting.co.uk/fec/.

28   Logitech Ltd. SightSpeed home page. [Online] Logitech Ltd, 2004–2009. [Cited: 25 July 2011]. http://www.sightspeed.com/.

[All links last accessed on 22 September 2011.]

Chapter 6 **Examples of technology in use**

Technology is being used in medical education in a wide variety of ways. Examples range from radio broadcasts used to supplement or provide a structure for face-to-face teaching sessions through to highly sophisticated, media-rich e-learning packages. Some of these approaches have a major positive impact for the learners and institutions that implement them. Others show no appreciable difference between the results of TEL and more traditional approaches. Even the latter approaches are still able to reap the benefits inherent to digital media effectively. This chapter aims to introduce some of the approaches being adopted worldwide and outlines common issues associated with each.

6.1 A Taste of Medicine

A Taste of Medicine [1] is a package produced by the e-learning unit at St George's medical school. It contains three modules. 'Getting started' is aimed at those considering applying for medical school. It is structured around common FAQs and includes a number of activities. Some of these activities are aimed at identifying personality traits in the learner that would indicate suitability to a career in medicine. Other activities compare a career in medicine against other career options that may be available to the learner. The module also includes video footage of first-hand experience of studying medicine from a student.

The second module is called 'Experiencing it'. It follows on from the previous module and aims to help prospective undergraduates to acquire first-hand experience of working in health care. The idea is that they will be in a

How to Succeed at E-learning, First Edition. Peter Donnelly, Joel Benson, and Paul Kirk.
© 2012 John Wiley & Sons Ltd. Published 2012 by John Wiley & Sons Ltd.

better position to make an informed decision about their career choice. This first-hand experience is also advised as a way to demonstrate their commitment during application for medical school. The module provides tips for making the most of voluntary and other work experiences. Some of these tips introduce the concept of reflective practice and the role it plays in learning and development. At this point, the module provides two options. The first is a link to a downloadable journal [2], which provides the framework necessary to record and reflect on work experiences effectively. The second is a link to the 'A Taste of Medicine Blog' [3], a free-to-use blogging tool that can be used to further support reflective practice and may also go some way to easing the transition to the use of online portfolios required further on in their careers.

The third module is called 'Scrubbing up'. It focuses on communication skills and includes the importance of effective and appropriate communication in a variety of personal and professional situations. The module is primarily designed to be used in a small-group setting; individual learners are advised to use the discussion points as points for reflection. It would be possible for individual learners to use a variation of the blog as a forum to discuss their thoughts. Implementing this without the accompanying assessment and moderation it would need is likely to produce limited results at best [4].

Figure 6.1 illustrates the graphical quality of this package. This high standard is maintained in all activities and media throughout the package.

This project shows that courses containing rich media can be very effective if they are underpinned with sound pedagogy. The use of rich media in this package creates a learning experience that is light-hearted, thought-provoking, lively and enjoyable. This experience not only prepares prospective applicants to St Georges, it creates the connotation that the institution itself is light-hearted, thought-provoking, lively and an enjoyable place to study. In short, it meets the learning objectives effectively and provides excellent advertising for the institution.

While rich media can be very effective, there are inherent dangers with using multimedia in e-learning packages. One is that if it is not carefully planned and underpinned by sound pedagogy, the media ends up overwhelming the message or activity rather than supporting it. This resource consistently uses multimedia to support and enhance the message that is being conveyed and to provide relevant learning and self-appraisal activities for the learner. This fine balance is not always easy to achieve.

Another inherent danger with using large amounts of multimedia in e-learning resources is that it can lead to the production of packages that will only work effectively over very fast Internet connections. 'Scrubbing

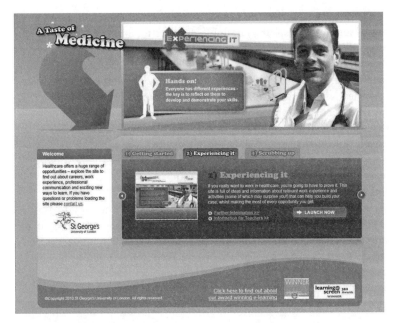

Figure 6.1 A Taste of Medicine

up' was aimed primarily at a UK-based audience so the media and its encoding are appropriate for this. However, if the target audience included sub-Saharan Africa, where there are very different conditions [5], another approach would need to be chosen.

6.2 Examples of innovative e-learning from developing countries

Large parts of the world do not have access to the kind of network infrastructure that is taken for granted in developed countries today. Until recently, most developing Commonwealth countries faced problems of slow Internet connections, few computers, an intermittent electricity supply, prohibitive costs, low information technology and communication (ITC) skill levels, social barriers and a lack of direction from policy makers. [5]

Some of the barriers experienced by developing countries are by no means unique to them. For example, a proportion of most developed countries is still restricted to low bandwidth or intermittent Internet connections in 2011, especially in rural areas.

Despite these barriers, there is a long history of TEL in the developing world and many inspiring examples of successful e-learning programmes. The following examples may not show cutting-edge technology in action or be directly related to medical education, but they do show innovative approaches to overcoming all kinds of barriers. They also show that technologies some consider to be antique are capable, in the right hands, of providing a high-quality educational experience to those who cannot access the alternatives. In a world full of new technologies, it is easy to forget that this is the ultimate goal of all forms of distance learning.

6.2.1 Zambia – the Interactive Radio Instruction (IRI) programme

The IRI programme [5 pp.42–5] began in July 2000. Its aim was to provide children who had no access to state schooling with the opportunity to follow the same syllabus and attain the same qualifications as those who had access to state schooling. The reasons for these children not being able to access regular state schooling included lack of places at state schools, distance and personal circumstances (parental deaths, pregnancies and other situations meant they had high levels of family commitments or low levels of support).

The IRI programme material consisted of interactive radio broadcasts, mentors and printed materials. The interactive radio programmes were broadcast to organised listening groups led by a mentor. The mentor would follow the pack while the students listened to the broadcast and would lead any activities outlined in the broadcast as per the training they were given and instruction from the pack.

The listening groups met before the broadcast was scheduled so that the mentor could recap on the previous work and hand out the previous day's assignments marks. After the broadcast, the students would stay to go through the exercises broadcast that day with the mentor. The mentor was also expected to train someone to take on their role in case they were not able to attend.

The results of the IRI programme are impressive. The programme started with 841 students enrolled in 28 listening groups; 1 year later there were 7782 students enrolled in 1153 listening groups. Some of these new listening groups were instigated and supported by the communities themselves after experiencing the benefits of groups in neighbouring communities. Another result of the programme is that parents and other adults asked to enrol. In 2002 there were adults ranging from 17 to 51 years old attending at two listening centres and going through the same syllabus as the children. Comparison of children who studied through IRI learning groups and those who attended state schools showed no significant difference in assessment scores, despite the fact that those who studied through the IRI programme covered the syllabus in half the time.

The IRI programme is not directly related to medical education or continuing professional development, but if we consider that clinical teams experience very similar barriers of distance from training centres, clinical commitments and lack of ICT infrastructure, it is highly probable that a similar model for short courses may prove to be just as effective for the professional development of clinicians in rural areas.

The IRI programme was launched over 10 years ago and there have been very significant global changes in ICT since then. Table 6.1 shows that Internet access in developing countries is experiencing rapid growth and a reduction in costs. Africa is well below the global average penetration rate of 30.2% but costs have been reduced by as much as 90% [6]. This will undoubtedly fuel further growth and competition will encourage providers to tap into more remote markets. This growth is encouraging, but many of the barriers to using TEL will still be present for the majority of developed and developing countries for some time to come.

Another major global change in ICT provision is that of the availability and cost of mobile devices. The digital education enhancement project (DEEP) illustrates how they can be applied to distance education with some surprising results.

6.2.2 DEEP

DEEP [8] is a collaborative project involving the Open University and a number of international partners. The aim of the original project was to investigate the use of ITC in teacher education across the developing world with the aim of:

- helping developing countries to provide flexible solutions to the problem of training enough teachers to meet the target set by UNESCO of providing universal basic education for all children by 2015;
- preventing developing countries making the same expensive mistakes that paved the way to ITC provision in the developed world;
- answering a number of research questions about using ITC in teaching and the professional development of teachers in developing countries [9 p.5].

DEEP's main focus was on how mobile computing and connectivity can be used to create community and school-based courses in sub-Saharan Africa. Trialling technological approaches is a primary goal of the project but it has been delivered with the knowledge that the true value in providing technology will only be seen if it is used to deliver resources that are pedagogically

Table 6.1 Usage, penetration and growth of Internet usage worldwide (Source [7])

World Internet usage and population statistics 31 March 2011

World regions	Population (2011 est.)	Internet users 31 Dec. 2000	Internet users latest data	Penetration (% population)	% Growth 2000–2011	Users % of table
Africa	1 037 524 058	4 514 400	118 609 620	11.4%	2527.4%	5.7%
Asia	3 879 740 877	114 304 000	922 329 554	23.8%	706.9%	44.0%
Europe	816 426 346	105 096 093	476 213 935	58.3%	353.1%	22.7%
Middle East	216 258 843	3 284 800	68 553 666	31.7%	1987.0%	3.3%
North America	347 394 870	108 096 800	272 066 000	78.3%	151.7%	13.0%
Latin America/Caribbean	597 283 165	18 068 919	215 939 400	36.2%	1037.4%	10.3%
Oceania/Australia	35 426 995	7 620 480	21 293 830	60.1%	179.4%	1.0%
World total	6 930 055 154	360 985 492	2 095 006 005	30.2%	480.4%	100.0%

sound, technically appropriate and firmly focused on the learning objectives that are to improve the professional practices of teachers.

The project took 12 pairs of teachers based in primary schools in Egypt and another 12 pairs based in Eastern Cape (one pair per school). These pairs would be given access to a variety of electronic resources for use in their teaching and a programme of professional development to help integrate the materials effectively. The materials provided included core professional development activities, incorporating a range of related lesson plans, printable activity cards, case studies, stories, video clips and links to websites. These were provided in the form of a CD-ROM and were also available for download via the project's website. E-books and an offline portfolio for recording student and teacher progression were also provided.

The exact technologies given for accessing the materials varied depending on what was most appropriate for each pair. An important aspect of selecting the right technologies was the decision to draw on those devices and technologies with which the teachers had already come into contact. While this led to some variation, all were provided with:

- a handheld computer, smartphone or PDA type device;
- a laptop with Internet access;
- a printer/scanner with ink;
- use of a video camera.

The devices were also equipped with the necessary software for accessing the materials and for generating new materials by the student or teacher. Over the course of the study, teachers and students did use the technology to generate new materials as Figure 6.2 shows. This particular example shows drawings made by the children to illustrate an African folk tale. The drawings were scanned into a computer and titles and captions were added. These were then used by the teacher as the basis for class discussion.

This particular activity took place less than 2 years after the technology and professional development had been put in place. Considering the reports of technophobia in teaching [9 p.59] and how profound the change is when introducing ITC into teaching and learning [9 p.108], it is remarkable that this happened so soon after the professional development and technology had been put into place.

The reason for this result is likely to be because the professional development was introduced alongside the technology. In developed countries, there is often an assumption that because a teacher or clinician knows how to use technology in their personal lives, they can easily use the technology appropriately in their role as a teacher; this is not a safe assumption to make. The skills used in e-moderation, for example, are more than a combination of

WORLD INTERNET USAGE AND POPULATION STATISTICS March 31, 2011						
World Regions	**Population (2011 Est.)**	**Internet Users Dec. 31, 2000**	**Internet Users Latest Data**	**Penetration (% Population)**	**Growth 2000-2011**	**Users % of Table**
Africa	1,037,524,058	4,514,400	118,609,620	11.4 %	2,527.4 %	5.7 %
Asia	3,879,740,877	114,304,000	922,329,554	23.8 %	706.9 %	44.0 %
Europe	816,426,346	105,096,093	476,213,935	58.3 %	353.1 %	22.7 %
Middle East	216,258,843	3,284,800	68,553,666	31.7 %	1,987.0 %	3.3 %
North America	347,394,870	108,096,800	272,066,000	78.3 %	151.7 %	13.0 %
Latin America / Carib.	597,283,165	18,068,919	215,939,400	36.2 %	1,037.4 %	10.3 %
Oceania / Australia	35,426,995	7,620,480	21,293,830	60.1 %	179.4 %	1.0 %
WORLD TOTAL	6,930,055,154	360,985,492	2,095,006,005	30.2 %	480.4 %	100.0 %

NOTES: (1) Internet Usage and World Population Statistics are for March 31, 2011. (2) CLICK on each world region name for detailed regional usage information. (3) Demographic (Population) numbers are based on data from the US Census Bureau . (4) Internet usage information comes from data published by Nielsen Online, by the International Telecommunications Union, by GfK, local Regulators and other reliable sources. (5) For definitions, disclaimer, and navigation help, please refer to the Site Surfing Guide. (6) Information in this site may be cited, giving the due credit to www.internetworldstats.com. Copyright © 2001 - 2011, Miniwatts Marketing Group. All rights reserved worldwide.

Figure 6.2 Material created by schoolchildren as part of DEEP. Reproduced from DEEP Impact: an investigation of the use of information and communication technologies for teacher education in the global south. http://www.open.ac.uk/deep/Public/web/publications/pdfs/ReportFeb2006.pdf © DEEP Project Team, Open University (OU)

email writing and the experience of leading a small-group activity offline. If guidance and training are not provided to make the transition effectively, it can lead to inappropriate use of technology, leaving clinical tutors and institutions concluding that online learning is not an effective teaching method for them.

There are other results from DEEP worth mentioning. The majority of the results [9 pp.59–89] are the kind expected from a project that is based on sound pedagogy and planning. Teacher confidence and practice were greatly improved along with their technical skills. The impact this had on their students was great and led to increased access to a wide variety of learning materials, acquisition of ITC skills, a better understanding of cultures outside their local context, higher motivation and, in turn, higher attendance and levels of academic achievement.

Other results of the study show that there were some key factors that influenced the major findings. One was that it is important for individuals to have ownership of the handheld devices used. This enabled them to experiment with different ways of using the devices at home before having to apply their ITC knowledge in a professional capacity. Encouraging peers to discuss technical issues and techniques, and communicating successes to the rest of the project groups were key factors in providing the support necessary for the growth of both ITC and professional development [9 p.19].

Another result was that when the costs of supplying and maintaining desktop and handheld computers were compared, handheld devices worked out as better value for money. The initial cost of refurbished desktop computers was cheap, but the cost of maintenance and repair was high. For handheld devices, the initial investment was high, but the fact that they were highly portable made them accessible to wider groups. Their durability in comparison to desktop or laptop computers meant that the cost of maintenance and repair offset the initial investment to a high degree [9 p.136].

DEEP and many other projects use CD-ROMs as the preferred fallback medium for distributing learning materials and courseware. The continuing drop in price of USB flash drives, laptops and mobile devices could mean that we are currently on the cusp of a new range of options for distributing high-quality e-learning resources in areas with little or no Internet access. It is currently possible to distribute a fully functional e-learning platform complete with courses on a USB stick. This approach can provide all pre-written learning materials and activities in a way that is completely independent of the Internet.

This approach does solve some problems but also resurrects one of the central challenges for any e-learning course design. This challenge is to provide the discussions and other social learning activities that are often used to help achieve and demonstrate mastery [10 p.222] and, in the case of DEEP, to provide invaluable peer support.

If we give a laptop access to the Internet via a mobile device, we open up many more possibilities. One possibility is to take a USB-based LMS and augment it so that the social learning tools and the progress each learner makes are connected to a central LMS. If this is done, we will have created a learning environment that is capable of delivering media-rich learning materials and supporting social learning with a vastly decreased dependency on the Internet. This approach could provide access to the kinds of course that have previously not been accessible to learners in some rural areas.

Mastery is not always the required outcome of distance learning, but if online social learning is required in remote areas with low bandwidth, new options are slowly becoming available. Even if the Internet is not an option in any form, there will still be some way for groups or individuals to communicate over large distances. These methods of communication may not be cutting-edge or even ideal, but in the right hands they can help provide access to relevant, high-quality learning experiences which, after all, are the ultimate aim of all distance and blended learning.

6.3 Examples from developed countries

6.3.1 Role of computer-generated 3D visualisation in laryngeal anatomy teaching for advanced learners – a prospective randomised study

This study by the University of Western Ontario [11] took a 3D model of the larynx constructed from images of cadavers and integrated it into a Web-based tutorial. This was then compared to 'standard' teaching comprising 2D images and a tutorial. Forty first- and second-year residents from surgery and anaesthesia took part in the study and were randomly assigned to one of two groups (n = 20). One group had access to the 3D model; the other was given the standard teaching. On assessment, there was no appreciable difference between the two groups, although residents preferred using the 3D model.

The fact that this study shows no difference between the two models is interesting. Both models take resources to create and deliver. In comparison to the 3D model, the standard teaching will take far fewer resources to create, but may need a tutor to be delivered. This means that the longer it is used, the more expensive it becomes.

The 3D model may take significantly longer and require specialist staff to create; however, once it is created, it can be delivered without intervention, at any time and to any amount of learners. This means the longer it is used, the more cost-effective it will be. It also means that learners are given the flexibility to take the 3D tutorial whenever they want and even repeat it if required. For an institution dealing with the demands of learners for flexibility, and limited staff resources for delivery, no difference is a significant result.

Even if the standard and 3D resources were identical in the way they were delivered, i.e. via the Internet and without intervention, the result of this study raises another interesting point.

Every medium has distinctive characteristics. If 3D models are used in some of the contemporary delivery mediums like Adobe Flash [12] or Unity [13], they can contain sound, respond to mouse clicks and do much more with 3D models than simply zooming and turning them on their axis. If a 3D model of the larynx used the medium to its full potential, it could be a resource that allowed simulated air to be visibly pushed by the lungs through the larynx to create sound. The model could then provide the means to relax and contract various muscles, providing a fully working model of the larynx. This would be very difficult to produce in any other medium and would provide illustration and a valuable learning activity in one package.

Having said this, the workings of the larynx have been taught very well using non-interactive 2D media and cadavers for many years so why invest in the development of a 3D model? One reason is this: good course design involves an awareness of the characteristics of each medium. E-learning technologists and instructional designers will take each point in the learning material and then choose the media and activity that are likely to facilitate it the best (depending on what is available to them). In some cases, the objective can be met using standard teaching; in others, the best way to meet the objective and facilitate deep learning may be to provide a fully working 3D model. If this is the case, a 3D model would be worth the investment.

The fact that this study showed no difference in assessment results for those who used 2D and 3D representations does not show a flaw in the study or in its use of 3D. Neither does it show that 3D is not a useful tool for learning anatomy. What it does show is that advanced learners can understand the anatomy of the larynx to the depth required by the assessment used in this study, irrespective of whether it is presented in 2D or 3D. Interestingly, it also shows that the learners taking part in this study prefer to learn using the 3D representation. Why they prefer the 3D option may shed further light on the performance of 3D in the teaching of anatomy.

If there is a take-home message from the studies in this chapter, it is this. If e-learning is planned and delivered with a sound understanding of the media, learners and pedagogy, all kinds of technologies can be used to create courses. They also demonstrate that these courses can be of a huge benefit to institutions and individuals.

References

1   Kenton Lewis, A Taste of Medicine. [Online] St George's, University of London Widening Participation Unit, 2010. [Cited: 29 June 2011.] http://www.tasteofmedicine.com.

2   Kenton Lewis, Journal to record work experience. A Taste of Medicine. [Online] St George's, University of London Widening Participation Unit, 2010. [Cited: 29 June 2011]. http://www.tasteofmedicine.com/experiencingit/journal.pdf.

3   Kenton Lewis, A Taste of Medicine Blog. [Online] St George's, University of London Widening Participation Unit, 2010. [Cited: 29 June 2011.] http://tasteofmedicineblog.com/.

4   Corich S, Kinshuk Dr, Hunt LM. Using Discussion Forums To Support Collaboration. Commonwealth of Learning. [Online] Commonwealth of Learning. [Cited: 29 June 2011]. http://www.col.org/pcf3/Papers/PDFs/Corich_Stephen.pdf.

5   Green L, Trevor-Deutsch L. Women and ICTs for Open and Distance Learning: Some Experiences and Strategies from the Commonwealth. Commonwealth of

Learning. [Online] Commonwealth of Learning, 2002. [Cited: 9 July 2011]. www.col.org/SiteCollectionDocuments/women%20and%20ICTs.pdf.

6 Lange P. Africa – Internet, Broadband and Digital Media Statistics (tables only). [Online] BuddeComm, 17 February 2011. [Cited: 10 July 2011]. executive summary outlining the growth of Internet usage in Africa. https://www.budde.com.au/Research/Africa-Internet-Broadband-and-Digital-Media-Statistics-tables-only.html?r=51.

7 World Internet Usage Statistics. [Online] Miniwatts Marketing Group, 2001. [Cited: 11 January 2012]. http://www.internetworldstats.com/stats.htm.

8 The Open University – UK. About DEEP. DEEP – Digital Education Enhancement Project. [Online] The Open University – UK, 2000. [Cited: 23 July 2011]. http://www.open.ac.uk/deep/Public/web/about/introduction.html.

9 Leach J, Ahmed A, Makalima S, Power T. Deep Impact: an investigation of the use of information and communication technologies for teacher education in the global south. Fuller-Davies Limited for Department for International Development (DFID), London, 2005. ISBN 1861927216.

10 Pear JJ, Crone-Todd DE. A social constructivist approach to computer-mediated instruction. Elsevier Science Ltd., Computers & Education 2002;38:221–231.

11 Tan, S. In: Z Kahn (ed.), Oral Presentations. Results from a comparative study of 3D model, plastic model and illustration by University of Western Ontario. doi: 10.1111/j.1365-2923.2011.04002.x Supplement s1: Wiley Blackwell, Medical Education 2011;45:32.

12 Adobe Inc. Rich Internet applications – Adobe Flash. Adobe.com. [Online] Adobe Inc, 2011. [Cited: 18 September 2011]. http://www.adobe.com/products/flashplayer/.

13 Unity. Unity Game Development Tool. [Online] Unity 3D. [Cited: 4 September 2011]. http://unity3d.com/unity/.

[All links last accessed on 30 September 2011.]

Chapter 7 **E-learning qualifications**

As we have seen in previous chapters and through our own experiences, technology is used broadly in two ways in an education and training context. In terms of enhancing the learning experience, we have seen many ways in which technology can facilitate new, rich, engaging and collaborative environments that serve and support learners in many and varied ways.

This chapter looks at how technology is used to facilitate learning via specific routes, which lead to formal qualifications, delivered online, in key areas for healthcare professionals, such as clinical, leadership, management, mentoring and legal. In this context, technology is used more widely to deliver learning, support learners, and provide course administration functions and management information to institutions.

Typically, in this context courses are supported using VLE technologies such as Blackboard or Moodle; these are environments that usually provide all the functions previously described. Users of these systems require credentials (user id and password), typically supplied by the institutions upon enrolment, in order to gain access to the learning environment.

Many lessons have been learned over the years following on, for example, from the experiences of the University of Athabasca [1], Open Universities Australia [2] and the Open University [3] in the UK in delivering learning at a distance.

There are challenges for institutions and for learners alike; these are in areas such as providing training for online tutors and providing timely support for synchronous and asynchronous communications – synchronous communications being particularly challenging where an international audience is involved, because differing time zones may mean learners/tutors

---

How to Succeed at E-learning, First Edition. Peter Donnelly, Joel Benson, and Paul Kirk.
© 2012 John Wiley & Sons Ltd. Published 2012 by John Wiley & Sons Ltd.

having an online appointment during unsociable hours. For learners there were early perceptions that pursuing a qualification via an electronic route was an easy option. This, of course, is untrue and while undertaking a course in an electronic environment provides key advantages in terms of flexibility, learning remotely at a pace, place and time of the learner's choosing to some degree, there are also substantial challenges for learners. They are 'out of class', for instance, with little peer pressure to engage. In fact, motivation to engage is key to success and institutions have set frameworks for 'keeping in touch' and encouraging learners to participate. The cost and commitment of enrolment on the course is usually a key step that helps learners to focus on the time commitment and whether they can commit to it.

The remainder of this chapter is a practical guide of a flavour of what is available in terms of e-courses that lead to a formal qualification. The market has grown hugely in the 5 years since 2006, and it is recognised that there will be high-quality offerings that are not mentioned here.

7.1 What to look for in an online course

7.1.1 First impressions

Your first contact may well be through a web search that directs you to a provider. Is their website well organised, inviting and customer-focused? Does it address your initial questions successfully – has the institution thought this through for you? Is there a structured search facility that facilitates your enquiry or do you have to trawl through endless pages to find what you are after? When were the pages last updated? This is an indication that the information you are viewing is current and can save you valuable time. Take the time to telephone and speak to someone; did you get through to a person easily (no protracted automated system) or did you have to leave a message? If so, did anyone get back to you? If the course is not provided in your country of origin/locality, check if there is a requirement to attend face-to-face sessions early in your enquiries as this may, of course, be potentially expensive/impractical etc. All this contributes to your perception of the quality of the provider and is an indicator of what you might expect in the future of your course.

You should also be able to find the information easily under the following headings (or similar).

Entry conditions
For example, here is a quote from 'Postgraduate Certificate in Prescribing for Allied Health Professionals' at Ulster University:

Prescriber candidates must be registered with the Health Professions Council and therefore already meet HPC standards for good health and good character.

Prescriber candidates must have a minimum three years full time experience (or equivalent) as a practising clinician and be deemed suitable by the employer to undertake the programme. Of these three years, the year immediately preceding application to the programme must have been in the clinical field in which the intention is to prescribe.

Employers must provide the University with evidence of a clean criminal records check on candidates conducted within the three years prior to admission.

Duration and mode of attendance

For example, attendance is required for 10 days; divided into three blocks of teaching; all further support is provided using the web. Is the mode semesters or terms?

Overview of the programme

The rationale for the course could be included here.

Structure and content

For example, the programme comprises 'X' compulsory 10-credit-point modules called 'Module A', 'Module B' etc. that in combination lead to the award of Postgraduate Certificate in 'Y'. The modules are usually taken over a 1-year period. The programme runs from January to May Module 'A', and September to December Module 'B' etc. each year.

Module 'A': attendance is required for 'Z' days divided into two blocks of teaching, with further support provided using Web-based resources.

Teaching methods and assessment

What teaching methods will be used? Is it interactive, using technology for support and small-group work around scenarios/cases, or someone standing up and talking? Delivery methods should address different learning styles and not be just a single mode – e.g. not just a lecturer talking. Do you have to attend face-to-face teaching sessions with the peer group?

How will assessment be achieved? Is it online or face to face, or a combination? What about exams, tests, portfolio presentation etc?

Professional recognition
Does the qualification lead to professional recognition in the field, e.g. recognised by Royal College of Medicine/Nursing/other national body?

Careers and postgraduate opportunities
What opportunities has the institution identified as a result of gaining a qualification in this area?

Contact details
The usual things you might expect are enrolment/administration contacts and perhaps, more importantly, a knowledgeable person with whom you can discuss your thoughts and queries about the course prior to enrolment.

Further information (for example, associated web links)
To facilitate access to course information, the remainder of the chapter is organised around the course categories of:
• clinical;
• leadership;
• management;
• mentoring;
• legal.

Each section contains the following subheadings to aid information presentation and consistent presentation: course title, provider, audience, qualification, overview and, where applicable, any special features.

The authors recognise there will be many other quality providers outside of those mentioned here.

7.2 Clinical courses

7.2.1 Master of Clinical Pharmacy [4]

Provider
University of Tasmania School of Pharmacy (UTAS).

Audience
The GradDipClinPharm and MClinPharm have been designed for registered pharmacists in any State or Territory of Australia, or registered in other countries, who wish to develop clinical and management skills and gain a postgraduate qualification in pharmacy.

This course would be particularly suited to those pharmacists who would like to offer pharmaceutical care or be better skilled to perform medi-

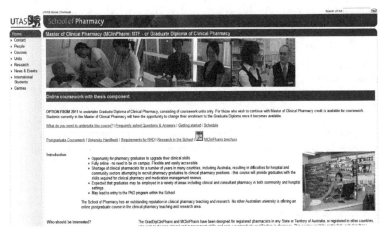

Figure 7.1 University of Tasmania School of Pharmacy. © University of Tasmania

cation reviews in patients' homes or nursing homes and residential care facilities.

Online delivery allows pharmacists who are unable to attend lectures to undertake postgraduate study off-campus. Pharmacists interested in research higher degrees can also use this degree as a foundation to further research study.

Qualification
Graduate Diploma ClinPharm and MSc ClinPharm.

Overview
UTAS states the objectives of the course as follows.

To develop the knowledge and skills of registered pharmacists leading to:
- a good understanding of the clinical features and therapeutic management of specific diseases;
- an ability to retrieve, interpret and apply published literature relating to pharmacy practice;
- the skills necessary to perform and report research projects relating to pharmacy practice;
- good verbal and written communication skills, to effectively communicate with other health professionals and patients.

Students will have a minimum of a bachelor's degree in pharmacy from the University of Tasmania or another university or tertiary institution which is deemed equivalent, and will be registered pharmacists. Where an undergraduate degree has been recently obtained, within the past 3 years, a minimum average grade of 60% obtained in the final 2 years of study would be required for entry. Appropriate postgraduation work experience of at least 2 years is also considered as a requirement for acceptance into these programmes.

Quote from former student

> *I did my research and found that UT was one of the best places to study in Australia and the School of Pharmacy had a good reputation. I didn't know much about Tasmania, but being an avid cricket fan, I had heard a bit about Hobart!*

7.2.2 MSc Clinical Education [5]

Provider
Edinburgh University.

Audience
The provider states:

> *The MSc in Clinical Education is for Health Care Professionals and Veterinary Practitioners, including doctors, nurses and professions allied to medicine, dental practitioners, and those involved with veterinary education. This extends to basic or social scientists who teach in medical, veterinary, dental or health care-education[sic].*

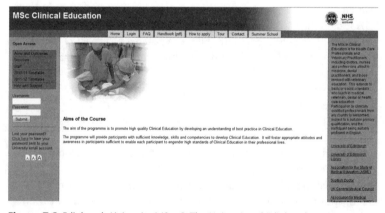

Figure 7.2 Edinburgh University MSc. © The University of Edinburgh

Participation by clinically qualified professionals from any country is welcomed, subject to a suitable primary qualification, and the participant being suitably proficient in English.

Qualifications
PG Diploma, PG Certificate or MSc in Clinical Education.

Overview
The following is an excerpt from what the provider currently offers:

The programme has been divided into a sequence of inter-related components, or 'Courses' that are compulsory for all students. There are 3 courses in each of the first two years which run on a 2-year carousel, followed by a Dissertation for completion at Masters level.

And:

Course material will be delivered online by formal teaching in the Forth Suite with additional resources and online tools accessed via the Clinical Education website and the University of Edinburgh Library Online. The first six weeks of each course start with one or more formal pre-recorded lectures which can be viewed online at a time convenient to the student. Later in each week there will be an online interactive, video-tutorial where students and a tutor work together in real-time. Normally this runs for one hour from 5-6pm or 6-7pm on Tuesday or Thursday evenings.[sic]

. . . Students are expected to attend the live tutorials sessions. Students also use self-directed learning, peer-discussion boards (online), peer presentations and other online activities to help them engage with the course materials.

7.2.3 Diploma in Practical Dermatology [6]

Provider
Cardiff University.

Audience
General practitioners.

Qualification
A Postgraduate Diploma Qualification in Dermatology.

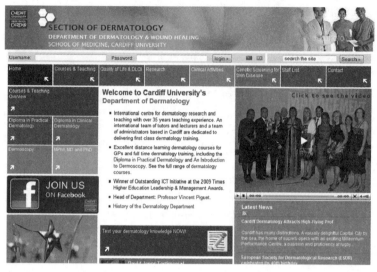

Figure 7.3 Cardiff University

Overview

The Diploma in Practical Dermatology (DPD) is a 1-year postgraduate distance-learning course for general practitioners who wish to gain expertise in the practical management of skin disease. It is a qualification for doctors wishing to establish themselves as GPs with a special interest in Dermatology or become clinical assistants.

Quoting the department:

> *This is a highly interactive online programme delivered through a state-of-the-art website. Through dedicated online tutorial support, discussion forums and online assessments, course participants become members of an enthusiastic and supportive online community of doctors with an interest in Dermatology. This environment allows collaboration, both academic and clinical, which extends beyond the life of the programme.*
>
> *The online content is supplemented by study meetings held at venues around the UK and Hong Kong.*
>
> *The DPD is one of only 27 courses in the UK accredited for Higher Professional Development by the Royal College of General Practitioners. Additionally it is a quotable qualification in Hong Kong and Singapore and is accredited in Australia.*

The department also offers an MSc qualification.

7.2.4 MSc in Practical Dermatology [7]

Audience
General practitioners.

Qualification
A Postgraduate MSc Qualification in Dermatology.

Overview
The MSc in Practical Dermatology launched in September 2009. The course begins with a 10-week block of online study to facilitate the development of study and research skills. Following the in-course formative assessment at the end of the 10-week study block, there is a 12-month window in which to submit the 20 000 word dissertation. After this time, a further 6 months is allowed in which any amendments may be made. The MSc is assessed by the submission of the dissertation.

Student quote

> The opportunity to do the Cardiff Diploma in Practical Dermatology came at the right time. Its 'on-line', Web Based, interactive format was ideal . . . [sic]

7.2.5 Postgraduate Certificate in Prescribing for Allied Health Professionals [8]

Provider
University of Ulster.

Audience
Allied health professionals.

Qualification
Postgraduate Certificate.

Overview
The programme comprises two compulsory 30-credit-point modules: Pharmacotherapeutics in Prescribing, and Prescribing in Practice, in combination leading to the award of Postgraduate Certificate in Prescribing for Allied Health Professionals and the professional award of Supplementary

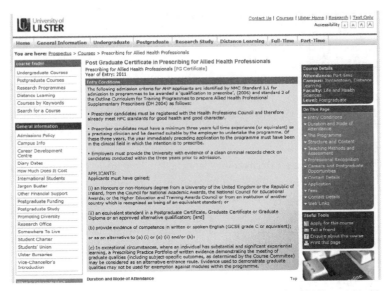

Figure 7.4 University of Ulster. © University of Ulster (Faculty of Life and Health Sciences)

Prescribing (for those professions eligible). The two modules are usually taken over a 1-year period. The programme runs from January to May (Module 1: Pharmacotherapeutics in Prescribing) and September to December (Module 2: Prescribing in Practice) each year.

Module 1: Pharmacotherapeutics in Prescribing – attendance is required for 10 days divided into three blocks of teaching; all further support is provided using the Web.

Module 2: Prescribing in Practice: Prescribing in Practice is delivered over 5 days – all further support is provided using the Web.

7.2.6 Edinburgh Surgical Sciences Qualification (ESSQ) [9]

Provider
University of Edinburgh.

Audience

> *The ESSQ programme is intended for those in the very early stages of their surgical training (pre-MRCS) and is based on the MRCS curriculum . . .*

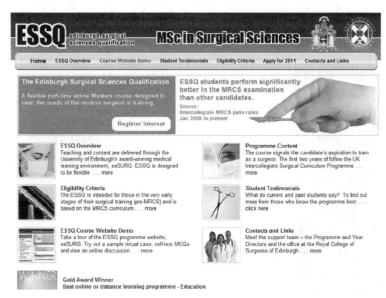

Figure 7.5 University of Edinburgh (ESSQ)

Qualification
MSc Surgical Sciences.

Overview
The provider offers the following information:

> *The programme is delivered through the University of Edinburgh's*
> *award winning medical virtual learning environment, eeSURG and,*
> *being online, is designed to give you the freedom to study flexibly . . .*
>
> *ESSQ consists of a modular programme building up by credit*
> *accumulation from certificate, through diploma and with the addition*
> *of a small research programme to a master's degree. The six modules*
> *leading to the postgraduate diploma cover the intercollegiate*
> *curriculum and consequently prepare students for the 'MRCS'*
> *examination and fees include an attempt at the MRCS exam. The*
> *third year MSc research project serves as an opportunity to develop the*
> *foundation of an academic career in surgery.[sic]*
>
> *The course follows the syllabus of the Intercollegiate Surgical*
> *Curriculum Programme . . .*

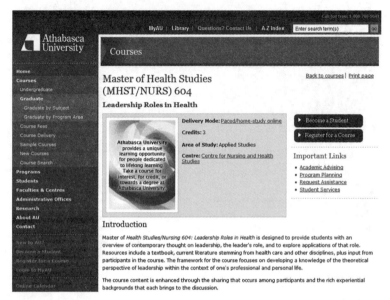

Figure 7.6 Athabasca University. © Athabasca University. www.athabascau.ca. Reproduced with permission

An online demonstration of what learners can expect is provided at http://demo.essq.ed.ac.uk/

7.3 Leadership courses

7.3.1 Master of Health Studies (Leadership Roles in Health) [10]

Provider
Athabasca University.

Audience
Healthcare professionals.

Qualification
Master of Health Studies.

Overview
Master of Health Studies/Nursing 604: Leadership Roles in Health is designed to provide students with an overview of contemporary thought on leadership, the leader's role, and exploring applications of that role. Resources

include a textbook, current literature stemming from health care and other disciplines, plus input from participants in the course. The framework for the course focuses on developing knowledge of the theoretical perspective of leadership within the context of one's professional and personal life.

The course content is enhanced through the sharing that occurs among participants and the rich experiential backgrounds that each brings to the discussion.

Students are strongly encouraged to seek additional resources beyond those identified and to share them with course participants. This mutual sharing and participation will ensure that each person gleans knowledge that will contribute to and enhance their personal leadership potential.

Special course features
In this course, you will access health-related websites worldwide. You will also participate in email and computer conferencing with other students. Students are expected to connect to an Internet service provider at their own expense.

Course goals
MHST/NURS 604 is designed to help you achieve the following course goals.
- Apply general leadership theory.
- Explore the competencies required to be an effective leader.
- Assess the relationship between leadership competencies and organisational effectiveness.
- Critically discuss selected topics related to leadership.
- Analyse personal experiences in light of relevant literature.
- Formulate an understanding of contemporary leadership thought.
- Critique your personal leadership capabilities identified during the course.
- Further develop your scholarly writing skills.

What is it like to be an AU student?
As an AU student, your student experience will be unlike that of students at traditional universities. You will probably take most or all of your courses through distance education, so the challenges and joys you will experience will be different. Here is an orientation to university-level study through AU. http://www2.athabascau.ca/students/index.php

7.3.2 MSc in Medical Leadership [11]

Provider
The Royal College of Physicians in association with Birkbeck College and the London School of Hygiene & Tropical Medicine.

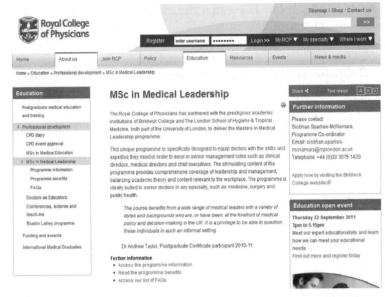

Figure 7.7 Royal College of Physicians. © 2012 Royal College of Physicians. *Reproduced by permission*

Audience
Doctors.

Qualification
MSc in Medical Leadership.

Overview
The Royal College of Physicians has partnered with Birkbeck College and the School of Hygiene & Tropical Medicine, at the University of London.
   Information offered by the provider:

> *This unique programme is specifically designed to equip doctors with the skills and expertise they need in order to excel in senior management roles such as clinical directors, medical directors and chief executives. The stimulating content of the programme provides comprehensive coverage of leadership and management, balancing academic theory and content relevant to the workplace. The programme is ideally suited to senior doctors in any specialty, such as medicine, surgery and public health.*

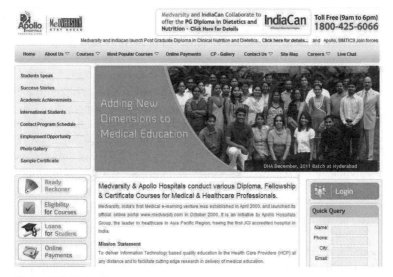

Figure 7.8 Medvarsity

7.4 Management courses

7.4.1 Healthcare Quality Management [12]

Provider
Medvarsity.

Audience
This Certificate programme in Healthcare Quality Management is specially tailored for healthcare professionals, both clinical and managerial including:
- quality managers . . . and all managers with a passion for quality;
- patient safety and risk management managers;
- staff involved in JCI and other accreditation processes;
- clinical directors and heads of departments;
- physicians and surgeons;
- heads of nursing and other senior nurses;
- clinical research managers;
- healthcare informatics and IT professionals;
- facilities, estates and support services managers;
- radiographers, laboratory, pharmacy and scientific staff.

Qualification
Successful candidates will be awarded the Certificate by Medvarsity, Apollo Hospital Educational and Research Foundation (AHERF) & Astron.

Overview
Healthcare services today are scrutinised, measured, evaluated and publicised as never before. An increasingly educated public expects to receive nothing less than excellent care and services and it must be the mission of every healthcare organisation to deliver that excellence. Quality improvement is the process of continually evaluating existing processes of care and developing new standards of practice and therefore has to be a core competency for every healthcare manager and clinician at every level of medical practice, be they in primary care clinics, acute hospitals, specialist centres of excellence or regulatory bodies.

Learning objectives
The Certificate Course in Healthcare Quality is designed to provide participants with a solid foundation of all the core elements of healthcare quality improvement. This course provides comprehensive coverage of the fundamental concepts, tools and management techniques through which quality management and improvement can be delivered in a healthcare setting.

It will therefore be invaluable, not only to those entering healthcare quality for the first time, but also for established healthcare managers needing an update of what is current in the field.

Course content
- Module-1: Introduction to Healthcare Quality.
- Module-2: Quality Management Tools and Theories.
- Module-3: Statistics in Quality.
- Module-4: Accreditation in Healthcare Quality.
- Module-5: Quality in Healthcare Organisations.
- Module-6: Patient Safety and Medical Errors.
- Module-7: Dashboards and Scorecards.
- Module-8: Past, Present & Future of Healthcare Quality.

Admission criteria
A Bachelor's degree from a recognised university.

Course duration
6 months with 2 days contact programme.

Course fee
Rupees. 23, 500/-.

Course highlights
- Course material developed by experienced specialists from Apollo Hospitals Group.
- Convenient to take the course as it is online anytime, anywhere learning with print support.
- No need to dislocate yourself from existing practice and place of work as the course is available both online and offline.

Course delivery
Our unique study approach enables you to balance your busy work schedule, social activities and travel so you can:
- study anytime, anywhere via the Internet;
- take your assessments online;
- get support in the form of books and articles;
- obtain an ID and password to access the course content and online assessments.

Certification
The student is required to complete all internal assessment tests. The final examination will be conducted at the end of the course.

7.4.2 Masters in Business Administration [13]

Provider
The Open University.

Audience
Practising managers aspiring to higher positions, normally aged 25 or over due to the requirement for managerial experience.

Qualification
Postgraduate Master's in Business Administration

Overview
The Open University has a long and distinguished track record in delivering quality education programmes, and this qualification is another of their highly regarded offerings.

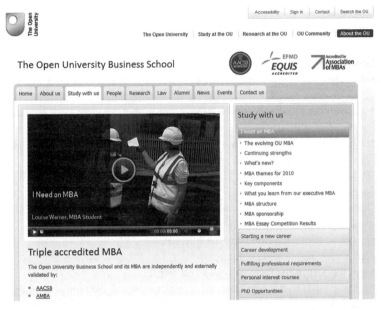

Figure 7.9 The Open University Business School. © The Open University

The following excerpt provides an overview of the course, but a visit to the website is a must, as there is much targeted information there:

> *This internationally-recognised MBA course is designed for practising managers aspiring to higher positions. The emphasis for your learning is directly rooted in management practice – the 'Master' in the degree title signifies your 'mastery' of the art and science of management. To achieve this level of capability the programme concentrates on strategic analysis, interdisciplinary skills, intellectual stimulation and independent judgement and builds these upon a solid foundation of core disciplines, including human resource management, organisational behaviour, accounting and finance, marketing and operations.*

One credit equates roughly to 10 hours of study and the Open University's MBA is a 60-credit programme.

7.4.3 Master of Business Administration (MBA) in Healthcare Management [14]

Provider
University of Phoenix, Arizona.

Audience
Healthcare staff with management experience.

Qualification
MBA.

Overview
The University provides this overview, but more in-depth information is available through filling out an online request form:

> *The Master of Business Administration (MBA) program prepares students in the functional areas of business allowing them to develop managerial skills necessary to be effective in a rapidly changing business environment. The program is based on current research of managerial competencies and graduate business standards as tested by existing national standardized graduate business examinations.*
>
> *Students in the Health Care Management Concentration will develop the managerial skills emphasized within the MBA required course of study in the context of challenges faced in the healthcare industry. They will be sensitive to legal, ethical, and social values in the management of healthcare resources. The Health Care Management Concentration is designed for students wanting to develop skills in the management of business operations in health care services organizations, health care related industries, small individual or group practices, and health insurance.[sic]*

The course requires at least 3 years of significant work experience.

7.5 General information on internationally available online MBAs

There are a number of online MBA programmes and 'MBAOnlineProgram' [14] ranks the current top five US providers as:

1 University of Phoenix;
2 Walden University;
3 Kaplan University;
4 Keller Graduate School of Management of DeVry University;
5 Northeastern University.

The MBAOnlineProgram states:

> *Employers today are demanding more education from their employees than ever before. An accredited online MBA degree will carry significant value in any organization's hiring and career advancement*

decisions. Plus, there is a direct correlation between higher salaries and earning and MBA.

7.6 Mentoring courses

7.6.1 Certificate in Mentoring [15]

Provider
The Institute of Counselling.

Audience
The Institute advises that the course is designed for:
- people who work with colleagues/clients etc. whose lives would be enhanced by a special kind of relationship where objectivity, honesty and trustworthiness are crucial;

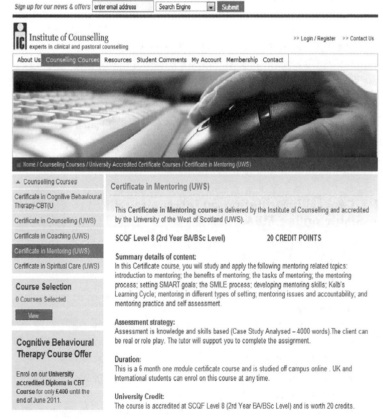

Figure 7.10 Institute of Counselling

- people who are specifically involved in the training and management of others;
- people who want to develop and enhance their career in mentoring;
- people who work in a caring/pastoral profession (social workers, nurses, teachers, ministers, etc.).

Qualification
Certificate in Mentoring, leading to a Diploma.

Overview
The Institute offers the following information about this course:

> *This tutor-supported distance learning course provides practical insights into the art of mentoring. The aim of the course is to equip you with the knowledge and skills to mentor others. This is achieved through providing insight into the process of mentoring and teaching the essential mentoring skills. Case studies, practical activities and assignments are included as key teaching tools.*
>
> *Mentoring is associated with positive personal and professional growth, career outcomes and development. It is a highly personal relationship that is creative, dynamic and intentional. Specifically, mentoring is where a more experienced individual (mentor) contracts to offer support, knowledge, interest and time to a less experienced individual (mentee). By doing this, the mentor enhances the mentee's personal and professional competency. The result for mentor and mentee is a greater sense of fulfilment, role definition and a more secure identity. This is beneficial to the individual, the organisation and the community. It can be seen that skilled mentoring can lead to tangible rewards in management development and practice.*

The course materials consist of 10 lessons, 5 tutor-marked assignments and a textbook. This is supplemented with suggested background reading.

7.6.2 Mentorship in Health Care Practice – online course (Level 3) [16]

Provider
Liverpool John Moores University.

Audience
Healthcare professions.

Qualification
Certificate of Mentorship in Health Care Practice – online course (Level 3).

Overview
The provider offers the following information:

> *This module will enable students to explore how to facilitate life long learning in others by developing their teaching, assessing and mentoring skills. Work based learning is the method used to help students achieve the module outcomes.[sic]*

Organisation of the course
The programme will be delivered during a 15-week academic semester. Students will only be required to attend an induction session, after which all coursework will be conducted via a virtual learning environment.
- Students will be supported throughout by the programme leader by email or telephone.
- Key texts will be available online.
- A postal library service will be available (students pay return postage only).

Course content
- Principles of learning.
- Experiential learning.
- Facilitation of learning.
- Teaching methods.
- Role modelling.
- The clinical learning environment.
- Principles of mentorship.
- Developing communication and working relationships with respect to students in practice settings.
- Principles of assessment.
- Relationship between clinical practice, education and research.

7.6.3 Certificate of Mentoring in Dentistry [17]

Provider
The Royal College of Surgeons of England, Faculty of General Dental Practice.

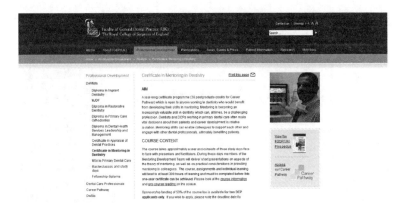

Figure 7.11 Royal College of Surgeons. © Faculty of General Practice (UK) 2012

Audience

The course is relevant to anyone working within dentistry. Applicants need to be computer literate; peer review and submission of formal assignments will be through a WBL system.

Qualification

Faculty of General Dental Practice (UK) Certificate in Mentoring.

Overview

The course takes approximately a year and consists of three study days face to face with presenters and facilitators. During these days, members of the mentoring development team will deliver short presentations on aspects of the theory of mentoring, as well as on practical considerations in providing mentoring to colleagues. The course, assignments and individual learning will lead to at least 300 hours of learning and must be completed before this 1-year certificate can be achieved. The remainder of the course is achieved through self-study and online learning.

7.7 Legal courses

7.7.1 Postgraduate Certificate/Diploma/MSc in Forensic and Legal Medicine [18]

Provider

University of Ulster.

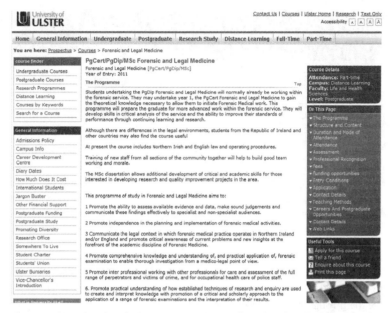

Figure 7.12 University of Ulster © University of Ulster (Faculty of Life and Health Sciences)

Audience
Applicants should hold an honours degree in a medical-, nursing- or law-related area from a recognised institution and will usually be a doctor or other qualified healthcare professional, manager or laboratory scientist, or be working in a forensic service position.

Qualification
Forensic and Legal Medicine Postgraduate Certificate/Diploma/MSc.

Overview
The provider states that:

> . . . students undertaking the PgDip Forensic and Legal Medicine will normally already be working within the forensic service. They may undertake year 1, the PgCert Forensic and Legal Medicine to gain the theoretical knowledge necessary to allow them to initiate Forensic Medical work. This programme will prepare the graduate for more advanced work within the forensic service. They will develop skills in critical analysis of the service and the ability to improve their

standards of performance through continuing learning and research.

The Postgraduate Diploma in Forensic and Legal Medicine will serve as preparatory study for The Royal College of Physicians, Faculty of Forensic and Legal Medicine (FFLM – RCP) MRCPath part 1 and part 2 examinations.

At present, the course includes Northern Irish and English law and operating procedures.

The MSc dissertation allows additional development of critical and academic skills for those interested in developing research and quality improvement projects in the area.

In terms of teaching and learning methods, the provider states the following:

> *The course uses a variety of teaching and learning methods. All teaching is by distance learning using internet-based teaching, multi-media resources, and online group discussion or by practical activity-based sessions and analysis of work-based material. The distance-learning course is delivered through the world-wide web, and in addition to the course team, distance learners are supported by e-tutors who act as mentors and provide personal and academic guidance.[sic]*

7.7.2 Masters in Medical Law [19]

Provider
University of Glasgow.

Audience
Lawyers, and particularly healthcare professionals.

Qualification
Masters/Diploma/Certificate in Medical Law.

Overview
An excerpt from the provider:

> *This programme provides a detailed account of medical law in Scotland and in England and Wales, including a rigorous exploration of the arguments around the law. The need to examine how law affects healthcare practice has become increasingly significant. This is due not*

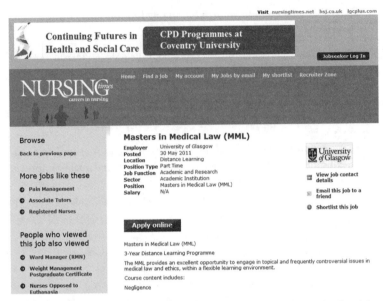

Figure 7.13 University of Glasgow. Reproduced from http://www.nursingtimesjobs.com/job/1280380/masters-in-medical-law-mml- © 2011–2012 EMAP Limited

only to patients seeking compensation for clinical injuries in ever larger numbers but also to frequent applications to the courts to settle issues relating to access to and the provision of appropriate treatment in complex and controversial situations, such as the withdrawal of treatment from severely disabled children. Recent legislation has changed the approach to adults with incapacity, organ transplantation, advance directives and assisted reproduction but controversy continues unabated around these and other subjects, including abortion and medically assisted suicide . . .

The MML is a part-time degree, taught over two years by online, interactive modules and attendance at two annual residential weekends. To provide maximum flexibility and choice, you can enrol for one year of the programme, leading to the award of PgCert in Medical Law, or for two years, leading to the award of PgDip in Medical Law, on successful completion of the relevant coursework.

References

1 Athabasca University home page, open and distance learning. http://www2.athabascau.ca/index.php.

2   Open Universities Australia, open and distance learning. http://www.open.edu.au/public/home.
3   The Open University, open and distance learning. http://www.open.ac.uk/.
4   University of Tasmania, Master of Clinical Pharmacy. http://www.pharmacy.utas.edu.au/mclinpharm.html.
5   University of Edinburgh, MSc Clinical Education. https://www.clinicaleducation.mvm.ed.ac.uk/.
6   Cardiff University, Diploma in Practical Dermatology. http://www.dermatology.org.uk/courses/dpd/dpd-overview.html.
7   Cardiff University, MSc in Practical Dermatology. http://www.dermatology.org.uk/courses/msc-practical/msc-practical-overview.html.
8   University of Ulster, Postgraduate Certificate in Prescribing for Allied Health Professionals. http://prospectus.ulster.ac.uk//course/?id=9707.
9   University of Edinburgh, Edinburgh Surgical Sciences Qualification (ESSQ). http://www.essq.rcsed.ac.uk/.
10   Athabasca University, Master of Health Studies (Leadership Roles in Health). http://www2.athabascau.ca/syllabi/mhst/mhst604.php.
11   The Royal College of Physicians in association with Birckbeck College and the London School of Hygiene & Tropical Medicine, MSc in Medical Leadership. http://www.rcplondon.ac.uk/education/professional-development/msc-medical-leadership.
12   Medvarsity, Healthcare Quality Management. http://www.medvarsity.com/HQM.aspx.
13   Open University UK, Masters In Business Administration. http://www3.open.ac.uk/study/postgraduate/qualification/f61.htm.
14   Masters in Business Administration, OnlineProgram top five list. http://www.mba-online-program.com/.
15   The Institute of Counselling (UK), Certificate in Mentoring. http://www.instituteofcounselling.org.uk/counselling-courses/certificate-courses/certificate-in-mentoring.
16   Liverpool John Moores University, Mentorship in Health Care Practice – online course (Level 3). http://www.ljmu.ac.uk/courses/cpd/76969.htm.
17   The Royal College of Surgeons of England, Faculty of General Dental Practice, Certificate of Mentoring in Dentistry. http://www.fgdp.org.uk/professionaldevelopment/dentists/mentoring.ashx.
18   University of Ulster, Postgraduate Certificate/Diploma/MSc in Forensic and Legal Medicine. http://prospectus.ulster.ac.uk/course/?id=7785.
19   University of Glasgow, Masters in Medical Law. http://www.gla.ac.uk/postgraduate/taught/medicallaw/.

[All links last accessed on 22 September 2011.]

Chapter 8 **Research**

8.1 Just in time, just enough and on the move

This chapter identifies and discusses various innovative technologies and approaches that have an online context, which is referenced. A good approach to using this chapter effectively is to open the reference link in a browser to experience the resource at first hand.

There is no doubt that developments and innovations in technology have provided new ways to deliver teaching and learning, and support learners in their quest for knowledge and skills.

Much of our modern technology has a basis in older forms of the same technology that has evolved over time; a good example of this is the mobile phone, which in principle relies on the same technology as the old 'wireless sets' of the 1920s.

Evolution in technology is interesting for a number of reasons and looking back, one aspect of technological evolution is the relatively short timescales over which significant advances were made. If we look, for instance, at electronics, which underpin the vast majority of modern technology, we see that the last 50 years have seen an evolution from the electronic 'valve' or 'vacuum tube' as it was known in the USA, to silicon chips in computer central processing units, which contain billions of transistors and provide the basis of modern-day computing.

The old 'valve' technology supported radio and early forms of television sets in the 1960s and 70s. In terms of teaching and learning, radio was a leap forward as it meant broadcast technology could disseminate information and support learners; probably the best-known examples are the Open

How to Succeed at E-learning, First Edition. Peter Donnelly, Joel Benson, and Paul Kirk.

© 2012 John Wiley & Sons Ltd. Published 2012 by John Wiley & Sons Ltd.

University UK, which delivered much content in the form of video-recorded lectures and demonstrations using television, Athabasca University Canada and the more recent Asia e-University.

If pace of change from the past is mirrored in the future, it may be that a diminishing healthcare workforce will face a fast pace of technological change, and the challenge will be to deliver and embrace TEL in a way that meets the needs of the workforce pressed to deliver service. There may be less time to engage in learning, so learning delivered 'just in time', 'just enough' (to meet the pressing current need) and 'on the move' will be crucial to the engagement of learners.

Miniaturisation of electronics-based technology has meant a revolution that, at its current point in support of teaching and learning, provides a plethora of gadgetry, proprietary systems and generic systems, which range from games-based, handheld, dedicated devices through to a vast range of computer software available for standard desktop-type computers and on to mobile technologies, which overlap with desktop computing but also have their own unique environments, advantages and dedicated systems that provide specialised learning environments such as simulation.

So what cutting-edge technology is there that supports teaching and learning? The remainder of this chapter looks at two key areas: virtual reality and simulation training.

8.2 What is virtual reality (VR)?

The term *virtual reality* may be used to describe environments that are heavily supported by computer hardware and software that provides a range of applications, which are immersive [1], highly visual, stereoscopic and 3D-oriented. Typically, VR is identified with head-mounted displays, gloves and data suits. These environments are becoming popular now in gaming circles with, for instance, the ability to play tennis with an online system by going through the physical motions of playing the game while holding the 'tennis racquet', which is a haptic device (device capable of providing physical sensory feedback to its user) linked to the computer system. It does not stretch the imagination too far, for example, to visualise these kinds of visual and sensory feedback systems in use in a surgical context to stitch a wound site [2].

Other VR environments include 'Second Life', which allows PC computer users to interact with an online virtual environment via inclusion of their avatar – a digital 3D-persona that is customisable in the virtual world – to create their online identity; e.g. in Second Life you can become a police officer, surgeon etc.

The remainder of this chapter looks at some examples drawn from VR and simulation applications in medicine.

8.3 Virtual reality systems in medicine

8.3.1 Overview

Key components of VR systems in the medical context include the following.

- Computerised graphics – these include 3D surface or volume rendering to give photorealistic representations of environments such as organs, operating theatres etc.
- Stereoscopic display systems – these are essential in order to provide realistic immersion into a virtual scene.
- Interaction devices and position monitoring – to facilitate integration and user immersion it is important to provide information about the actual physical status of the observer while they interact. e.g. with virtual surgical instruments.
- Force or tactile feedback – an important source of information when interacting with the virtual environment. The forces have to be transmitted to the user if immersion in a virtual scene is to be achieved with a high degree of realism, e.g. when stitching a wound in a VR environment, a user would expect to feel the pressure of the tissues and tension of the stitching material as the process progresses.
- Other sensory feedback may include olfactory and auditory.

8.3.2 Simulation systems in VR

What are simulation systems?

Simulation systems are a particular branch of VR, probably best known in medicine as the life-size patient simulator; however, many other forms of simulation are currently available that apply to specific medical specialties.

8.4 VR in obstetrics and gynaecology

Ultrasonographer trainees need to develop a mix of cognitive skills and eye–hand movement coordination so they acquire the skills and experience to obtain appropriate images by manipulation of the ultrasound probe; they also need to recognise and interpret ultrasound images in order to make a diagnosis.

The training required is time and resource intensive, and requires repeated patient contact in the clinical setting. Until recently, this training was acquired through 'hands-on' experience with ultrasound machines and real patients in a highly supervised environment.

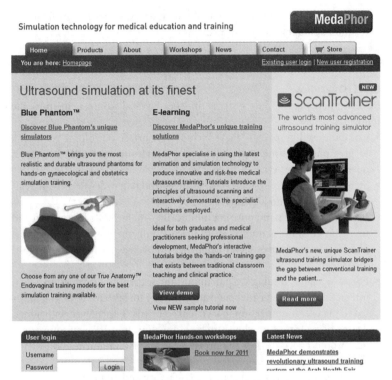

Figure 8.1 ScanTrainer ultrasound simulation. © MedaPhor Ltd

As a result, trainees could only practise and learn when these training resources were available.

One example of a VR system that seeks to address the situation outlined above is provided by Medaphor [3], a company which specialises in obstetrics and gynaecology training.

Medaphor's ScanTrainer product is designed to simulate the endovaginal exam, and by accurately mimicking the feel and imaging characteristics of an actual clinical exam, users of this system can develop and perfect the skills necessary to utilise ultrasound in a clinical environment..

Features of this VR are as follows.

- It uses a haptic probe to provide realistic sensory feedback to the user.
- It bridges the gap between conventional training and contact with real patients to improve the quality of learning prior to patient exposure.
- It combines photorealistic animation with haptic simulation techniques to provide a realistic feel to the simulation.

- Curriculum-based interactive learning modules are integrated with the simulation to provide a blended approach.
- The systems are designed to provide sophisticated ultrasound learning in a non-clinical environment, solving the current resource conflict between the provision of clinical service and the need to train.
- It may be used self-directed.
- The system provides a variety of anatomy and pathology programmes.

8.5 Life-size patient simulators

These devices are portable and provide an advanced patient simulation context. They typically provide realistic anatomy and clinical functionality. The sophisticated software and haptic and other sensory feedback systems can provide challenging care scenarios that test students' clinical and decision-making skills. Simulators of this kind have become available as a direct result of miniaturisation of technology, development in artificial intelligence and 'heads-up' display contexts developed particularly in the military arena. If we think of the parallels with the miniaturisation of computers and the branching evolution of computing power into handheld devices such as PDAs and phones, it seems likely that continued miniaturisation will take life-size patient simulator environments into more realistic field-based scenarios that embrace the environment in which treatment may need to be administered – e.g. a simulated road traffic accident.

Laerdal's SimMan [4] is an example which provides the following benefits to learners.

- Educational effectiveness – the system provides highly realistic patient simulation training experiences for the practice of teamwork, leadership and communication skills.
- Multidisciplinary teamwork – it facilitates training of a range of healthcare professionals encompassing all areas of patient care.
- It facilitates practice on uncommon scenarios – the unusual cases that learners may face in real life.
- Anatomically realistic – it enables a wide range of emergency medical interventions to be practised.

Features of these VR types include the following.

- Typically they provide full-scale patient simulation that can facilitate relevant advanced life support (ALS) skills and scenarios.
- Manikins are comprehensively interactive, giving immediate realistic feedback to interventions.
- They may include a simulated patient monitor with touch-screen technology.

- Typically they include the facility to preprogram scenarios and save a set of user-defined scenarios/cases.
- An instructor's panel controls how the physiological parameters will change over time.
- They may provide software for generating automatic debriefing, based on an event log synchronised with video pictures, to provide detailed feedback on performance to learners.
- Instructors can change parameters behind a two-way mirror as the scenario evolves.

8.5.1 Advantages

These simulations provide opportunities for learners and teachers to explore difficult and challenging situations in a multifaceted, controlled environment. Scenarios are dynamic and typically evolve as treatment progresses. Simulation scenarios embrace wide-ranging situations from a relatively uncomplicated bedside encounter on the ward to a road traffic accident in A&E. Significant advantages for learners are obtained from reflection and debriefing.

8.5.2 Disadvantages

The generic disadvantages of these experiences are outlined below (see Second Life disadvantages).

8.6 Other simulation examples

In their paper entitled 'The Use of Surgical Simulators to Reduce Errors' [5], the authors describe the use of a simulator for endoscopic sinus surgery (ESS). They state:

> *The emphasis on patient safety in the operating room has focused historically on the numerous supportive functions involving devices, medications, staffing, and administrative procedures, but rarely on the surgeon's technique and performance.*

They also note:

> *Given that competence and safety are of paramount importance, the objective measure of a resident's progress is a critical factor and one that his or her teachers address diligently.*

Traditional face-to-face training and skills acquisition in the workplace is naturally dependent upon the patients of the attending surgeon and their presenting situations; the authors explain the difficulty of continued competency in unusual cases (which occur infrequently), and gaining the necessary competences surrounding them. They describe a simulator for ESS and its benefits:

> *Computer-generated surgical simulation affords the ability to create an environment that imitates the real surgical world without inherent risk to the patient, and the technology serves to overcome many of the limitations of current training approaches. Procedures can be repeated until proficiency is achieved, techniques can be refreshed or learned anew, the variability of case-mix (or lack thereof) can be overcome, and competency can be assessed by certifying boards or hospital accreditation panels, prior to taking a single patient to the operating room. Moreover, new devices can be tested in a simulated environment, and new procedures can be rehearsed or improved, without exposing patients to potential risk of harm.*

So we see here further examples of why simulation is perceived as a valuable component in training. A video link to such a simulator is provided in the references [6]

8.7 Whole-heart modelling

In a recent paper [7], the authors describe developments in cardiac simulation:

> *Recent developments in cardiac simulation have rendered the heart the most highly integrated example of a virtual organ. We are on the brink of a revolution in cardiac research, one in which computational modelling of proteins, cells, tissues, and the organ permit linking genomic and proteomic information to the integrated organ behaviour.*

8.8 Telling stories: understanding real-life genetics [8]

This resource led the way in setting real-life patient stories within an education framework. Patient stories are available as video archives and a sophisticated search facility allows retrieval according to user needs and contextual criteria. A number of sample usage frameworks are provided to help educators deliver genetics education sessions.

8.9 Second Life VR

Second Life [9] is part of a group of web technologies called Web 2.0, which feature immersive, graphically and interactively rich environments.

It was created by Linden Lab in 2003 and is a free, 3D virtual world where digital personas travel, work, play and socialise through chat rooms and other, often photorealistic and interactive online gathering places.

Millions of users enter Second Life regularly to meet friends, socialise, buy and sell etc. Companies, universities and other organisations increasingly have an online presence in Second Life.

Wider examples of Web 2.0 are Facebook, Flickr and Twitter. This section looks at some 'Second Life' offerings.

8.9.1 VR in addiction therapy [10]

The following quote from the 'Medicine meets VR' conference in 2009 gives a flavour of the Second Life environment:

> *Use of VR in Addiction Medicine: During the exposure, participants are encompassed within a sensory isolation apparatus, including a 32 LCD monitor and a surround-sound audio system. Participants interact with the specially created virtual world in Second Life, run from a standard Dell PC, using a simple gaming remote control. An additional monitor is placed outside of the apparatus for outside observation.*

This resource was created through the work of the Neuropsychiatric Institute at UCLA. It demonstrates how, through a blended approach, such systems can add value to learning programmes. A computer workstation with a 32-inch monitor, video game controller and surround-sound audio system has provided an immersive experience for participants in the virtual environment, while they remain in the safety of a clinical setting.

Features of this VR
Participants experience the VR environment from a first-person perspective and can control their avatar with a handheld video game remote.

Participants may explore a wide range of inanimate cues (e.g. pipes, lighters, bags of meth, syringes, lines of meth) and encounter animated cues (e.g. avatars smoking, snorting and injecting meth) within a native context.

Participants are prompted by audio clips to interact with the inanimate cues (e.g. 'Click on the pipe if you want a hit.'), which allows the participant to engage in drug-taking behaviour.

Changes in participants' self-reporting of subjective responses, e.g. 'How much do you crave meth right now?', and physiological state, e.g. heart rate and blood pressure are closely monitored at regular intervals during each exposure to determine the effects of this novel method of cue exposure compared to traditional methods.

Evaluation: the authors state 'Future studies will further record and analyse participants' behaviour and movement within the virtual environments to assess the efficacy of treatment.'

As with any new and innovative education/training intervention, appropriate evaluation of the project should be provided. It is vital that evaluation is built into the project from the outset, so that key opportunities for evaluation criteria creation and measurement are not missed. Quite often such interventions take time and require financial resources to start up, so evaluations that show the added value, if any, are important for the resource to be integrated into learning programmes and also in order to inform future development of the resource.

8.9.2 Further examples

At Imperial College London [9], the question 'Can Second Life help teach doctors to treat patients?' was asked.

Medical students using the Imperial application of Second Life can navigate a full-service hospital where they carry out a typical scenario – see patients, order X-rays, consult with colleagues and make diagnoses.

Jeremy Bradley at CNN observes:

> Prospective doctors are treating virtual patients in Second Life, the
> Internet world where users interact through online alter egos called
> avatars. The third-year med students are taking part in a pilot
> program for game-based learning, which educators believe can be a
> stimulating change from lectures and textbooks.

In this application, students sit at computers and enter the virtual Second Life hospital as an avatar. The grounds are designed to resemble Imperial College London, and signs point the students toward the respiratory ward.

Students are allowed to collaborate only through their avatars.

The scenario continues:

> After the avatars enter the computer-generated hospital, they check in
> at a reception desk, put on an access badge, and then stop by Professor
> Martyn Partridge's office to get their assignment…If students forget to
> wash their hands before visiting a patient, their investigation is halted.
>
> Then students enter a patient's room and their work begins. Because
> their assignment takes place in a respiratory ward, they can access
> recordings of real-life patients' breathing to help with their diagnoses.
> And if students decide that X-rays are needed, they can stroll down to
> the radiology department and order them.

All these steps are designed to reinforce lessons about responsibility and hospital protocol.

'This sort of research is vital if we're going to make sure tomorrow's doctors are as well-trained as you and I want them to be,' said Partridge, Professor of Respiratory Medicine at Imperial College London.

Second Life at the Ann Myers Medical Center [11] (AMMC)

Aims to assist students to become more proficient in initial exam history and physicals; to become more proficient in the analysis of MRIs, CTs and X-rays. You can join to take part in the first medical simulation.

The Second Life environment relating to AMMC virtual training for doctors, nurses and students is also described in a YouTube [12] video.

Heart murmurs [13]
This is another example of educational possibilities in Second Life as you visit a treatment centre and listen to cardiac murmurs.

The Gene Pool [14]
This is a good-quality genetic educational place in Second Life. There are quizzes, animations and the opportunity to wear your favourite chromosome-patterned tee-shirt.

Virtual Neurological Education Centre [15]
This provides an online virtual environment for training and demonstrating virtual experiences of neurological disorders.

Medical Library at Health Info Island [16]
PUBMED searches from Second Life: find people at the Medical Research Desk or at the Consumer Health Information Desk. This is a growing medical virtual community.

Centers for Disease Control and Prevention [17]
The National Review of Medicine [18] indicates that the centers are one of the early adopters. They consider Second Life as an educational opportunity to access large audiences.

Wheelies @ Second Ability [19]
This is a place for people with disability. You can try out what it is like to use a wheelchair.

8.9.3 Advantages

Learners can practise in safe, controlled and measured environments. A variety of situations can be presented, some of which the learner may experience relatively infrequently in their everyday practice. The environments are engaging, potentially competitive and challenging.

8.9.4 Disadvantages

The generic disadvantages of these experiences may be outlined as follows.

- The user has a nominal experience that, although it supports and upskills the user, they can walk away from without consequence; so the realities of pressure of work, non-ideal conditions, tiredness and the pressure of needing to get it right first time with a real patient are not there.

References

1 Immersive learning. http://www.youtube.com/watch?v=R3WLJq5BucM.

2 VR environments – a useful general article on VR in medicine. http://www.ncbi.nlm.nih.gov/pmc/articles/PMC1129082/.

3 Medaphor endovaginal training system. http://www.scantrainer.com/.

4 SimMan. http://www.laerdal.com/gb/doc/86/SimMan?docid=1022609. SimMan youtube video. http://www.youtube.com/watch?v=gBNGKZnHVHc.

5 The use of surgical simulators to reduce errors. http://www.ncbi.nlm.nih.gov/pubmed/21250030 and http://www.ncbi.nlm.nih.gov/books/NBK20604/#top.

6 Endoscopic sinus surgery video. http://www.howcast.com/videos/229847-Virtual-Sinus-Surgery-Simulator.

7 Imperial College London. http://articles.cnn.com/2009-03-30/tech/doctors.second.life_1_second-life-medical-students-virtual-hospital?_s=PM:TECH.

8 Telling stories: Understanding real-life genetics. http://www.tellingstories.nhs.uk/.

9 Second Life. http://secondlife.com/.

10 VR in addiction therapy – 'Second Life'. http://www.etc.ucla.edu/research/projects/Meth-Apartment.htm.

11 Ann Meyers Medical Centre – Second Life examples. http://scienceroll.com/2007/06/17/top-10-virtual-medical-sites-in-second-life/.

12 AMMC training. http://www.youtube.com/watch?v=QnTzgon-Wto.

13 Heart murmurs. http://scienceroll.com/2007/06/17/top-10-virtual-medical-sites-in-second-life/.

14 The gene pool. http://scienceroll.com/2007/06/17/top-10-virtual-medical-sites-in-second-life/.

15 Neurological disorders. http://scienceroll.com/2007/06/17/top-10-virtual-medical-sites-in-second-life/ and http://slurl.com/secondlife/Lost%20Islands%20NW/46/80/200.

16 Virtual library. http://scienceroll.com/2007/06/17/top-10-virtual-medical-sites-in-second-life/ and http://slurl.com/secondlife/Healthinfo%20Island/65/68/323.

17 Centers for disease control and prevention. http://scienceroll.com/2007/06/17/top-10-virtual-medical-sites-in-second-life/.

18 National review of medicine 2007. http://www.nationalreviewofmedicine.com/issue/2007/03_30/4_advances_medicine_6.html.

19 Wheelies at second ability http://scienceroll.com/2007/06/17/top-10-virtual-medical-sites-in-second-life/ and http://slurl.com/secondlife/Showashinzan/26/116/301.

[All links last accessed on 30 September 2011.]

Chapter 9 **Looking towards the future**

It could be argued that looking towards the future is best achieved by identifying and exploring trends rather than trying to second-guess (and inevitably get it wrong). A useful starting point is to look at what has happened in the technology-enhanced learning context in the last 5 years (since 2006). Other chapters in this book give some insight into this, but it may be useful to summarise and explore key aspects of 'what has happened recently' in order to look to what may happen in the future.

9.1 The recent past

The future will to some extent be built on the recent past and the following gives us some ideas of key milestones that will likely be useful building blocks in future.

- Time to market for multimedia resource construction has been significantly reduced.
- Multimedia authoring has become much easier with tools such as Camtasia and Captivate widely available.
- Mobile technologies have 'come of age' and now provide powerful devices and networks that make them highly usable in a teaching and learning context.
- Flash Player has become widely adopted as the Web-based audio/video streaming standard (with the notable exception of Apple).
- Learning management systems such as Moodle and Blackboard have become widely used as information repositories, and delivery and assessment tools in schools, colleges and the higher-education context.
- The emergence of social learning networks [1].

How to Succeed at E-learning, First Edition. Peter Donnelly, Joel Benson, and Paul Kirk.

© 2012 John Wiley & Sons Ltd. Published 2012 by John Wiley & Sons Ltd.

Given these milestones, how might the future unfold in terms of technology?

It looks highly likely that people's engagement with mobile technology will provide opportunities to deliver education and training 'just enough, just in time, and on the move'. The concept of personalised learning has been around for some time and indeed in the past presented significant challenges to teachers in a face-to-face environment – how do you tailor what you are delivering to meet the needs of a mixed-ability audience? Given our modern technological environment, a key development will doubtless be 'personalised learning' in an electronic context, but this will require evolution of some present-day technologies. Learners would be able to access multimedia content from work-based information systems 'just in time'. Collaborative learning will evolve and individual learners will contribute their own content using mobiles devices. The following will be required to support mobile learning.

- Mobiles need to be predicated on Android-type open-source interfaces (Moodle gives an insight into the popularity of open source).
- Tablets such as the iPad (there will be many others to choose from) will become much more functional.
- Learning management systems will evolve to incorporate newer tools in order to support the personalised-learning context and will include:
  - learning management technology for blended or informal learning;
  - learning management technology for compliance training;
  - social learning technology;
  - informal learning measurement/assessment.
- Authoring tools will become easier for non-technical people to use; a 2011 example is Zebra [2] from the authors of 'Authorware'.
- Game-based learning will continue to develop and products such as 'Unity' [3] which is now available for Android phones, will further empower those wishing to embrace this field.
- There is a drive to optimise learning and this will continue with integrated approaches to workplace-based learning, simulation, technology-enhanced learning and face-to-face learning.

Personalised-learning needs' assessment will be key to mobile technologies' capability to deliver appropriate learning for learners. BMJ Learning has pioneered this concept as a Web-based tool with doctors in Wales, UK. Such needs' assessment could take the form of a mobile application that searches out up-to-date information based on personal preferences and just-in-time learning needs for the workplace.

9.2 Why is 'computing power' important and how is it defined?

An interesting enigma is provided by Moore's law [4]; Gordon Moore is an Intel cofounder, and the law describes a long-term trend in the way computer hardware capability changes with time. Electronic hardware functionality is essentially made up of devices called transistors and these are manufactured as integrated circuits. Moore's law describes the fact that every 2 years, the number of transistors that can be placed in an integrated circuit doubles. This trend has been in evidence for more than half a century and is expected to continue perhaps until 2020 or later.

The point of this is that the capabilities of many digital electronic devices are strongly linked to Moore's law, as essentially we get more miniaturisation and more power in our devices (such as mobile 'phones).

9.3 Past trends informing future trends

Tom Vander Ark was the first Executive Director for Education at the Bill & Melinda Gates Foundation. In a 2011 article [5], Vander Ark cites 'Megatrends' [6] and predicts the following future 'Megatrends'.

9.3.1 Personal technology

Expanding access to personal digital learning is one of the most important world shaping megatrends. People, schools, states, and countries that embrace digital learning will, as President Obama has urged, 'win the future'. As Naisbitt pointed out, '. . . access to personal communication technology is transformational – just ask one of the 650 million people in India who have cell phones'. [sic]

9.3.2 Personal digital learning

With broadband access, it is possible for anyone anywhere to learn almost anything. Informal learning opportunities are exploding and right behind them are low cost online credentialing options that will expand access to quality secondary learning to the 500 million young people that lack access today. Broadband, cheap tablets, open content, and inexpensive blended schools will rapidly expand access to post secondary learning and information economy careers in emerging economies.

Brian Kuhn [7] proposes 'Technology is a game changer for learning':

I know, it's not about the technology. We all say it. But, I think we may be kidding ourselves. Look around and you'll see technology changing and challenging almost everything. It makes things possible that weren't necessarily even a thought before. Think about the iPhone – did the millions upon millions of people 'know' they needed it before it was? Our modern tools, conveniences, and inventions today would not be possible to design, engineer, or produce without sophisticated technology.

Many would argue that the technology is there to support the learning and that pedagogy (the science of learning) must drive the technology requirement; so we decide which technology would be best suited to what we are trying to do.

Kuhn continues:

For schools and classrooms there is often a debate about technology as a tool, technology as a skill, or even that there is no need for it. We often suggest that technology is a nice to have but real teaching and learning can continue on without it as it always has. In light of all the writing and discussion about 21st century learning, personalized learning, etc., is this really still the case?

This is, of course, a very interesting point and any future for teaching and learning we can think of would be difficult to envision without a heavy technology component.

Kuhn concludes:

More now than ever, educators need to be incorporating and modelling the effective use of technology in their teaching. They need to guide students in their use for learning and ensure they gain the 21st century skills necessary to be fully literate.

Kuhn's web article describes a 'touch-screen vision' for teaching and learning and shows a very interesting video clip [8] on touch-screen technology:

. . . We were reviewing classroom design characteristics. We are including a lot of glazing (windows) to create an open and transparent learning space. I asked about the cost and technical difficulty of replacing the windows with digital multi-touch material once such options were available and affordable – it may not actually be that difficult . . . Imagine being able to, on demand, have these windows be transparent (like a window) or a scene from history or some other

place on earth to match the current lesson. Also, the window could be a multi-touch interactive video surface – students could speak and interact with other students around the world, relevant to their current lessons. I see the above video (cited in the article) as being a feature of these windows, perhaps well before 2020 . . .

Sharples [9] describes the concept of a handheld learning resource (HandLeR). Characteristics of this personalised, learning needs system are described:

We have given our HandLeR the role of a 'mentor'. A mentor system can act as a companion to a young learner (a partner in games, for example); it can suggest ways of studying and set up systems for organising resources and remembering ideas and events; it can provide long-term guidance on developing skills, particularly where the mentor could have direct access to the technology needed for performing the skill (such as the Worldwide Web, or a digital camera); it can act as a learning assistant in performing tasks or solving problems, by suggesting new strategies and solutions; for professional development it can store and abstract information from cases (such as medical images) and support experiential learning. A computer-based mentor need not reside in a single piece of hardware; it might migrate across different physical devices, but retaining its persona and knowledge of the learner.

Such a personalised-learning manager would need the 'means to store, organise and retrieve cases, events, and knowledge structures'. Sharples describes how software is dissociated from the hardware platform so that lifelong learning is facilitated (i.e. there is no hardware dependence so as technology becomes obsolete, this is not a problem).

9.4 Experiments involving neurosurgical implants

Not wishing to become too MATRIX-like (for those fans of the Wachowski brothers' sci-fi films), a unique experiment performed by Professor Kevin Warwick of the University of Reading [10] may inform an intriguing future interface between humans and machines. In 2002, an electrode array 'was surgically implanted into the median nerve fibres of the left arm of Professor Kevin Warwick. The operation was carried out at Radcliffe Infirmary, Oxford, by a medical team headed by the neurosurgeons Amjad Shad and Peter Teddy'. The experiment allowed Professor Warwick to control an artificial hand and the electronics measured the nerve signals to achieve this.

Google Goggles in action

Click the icons below to see the different kinds of objects and places you can search for using Google Goggles.

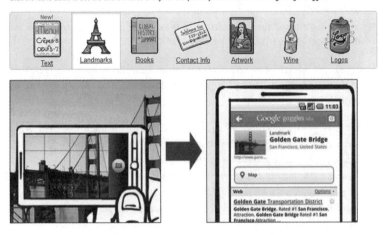

Learn more in the Mobile Help Center or ask questions in our Help Forum.

©2011 Google - Terms of Service - Privacy Policy

Figure 9.1 Google Goggles

This example perhaps gives us an insight into how technology and human interaction may develop in the future.

9.5 Ongoing development in mobile technology

At the time of writing, '4G technology' [11] is expected to bring superfast Internet connectivity to mobile devices. An innovative example of how improved performance facilitates more powerful searching is provided by 'Google Goggles'.

Google Goggles facilitates searching using pictures taken with phones to search the web without using text. Users open the application, take a picture and wait for the results. The application works with a range of products, such as books, DVDs, landmarks, logos, art, barcodes and text.

Google advertises this product with a tourist in a restaurant who takes a picture of the menu using their phone. Google returns a translation of the menu into English.

Further development of this product will widen its ability to recognise many objects/situations and one can easily imagine developments such as this in a medical context.

Google Goggles is an example of an 'Android app' (an application which runs on the open-source Android phone operating system), and many of these will become available through this open-source avenue. The power of open source is encapsulated in the name – the source programming code that is used to define the application is freely available without cost. This enables any interested party to contribute, change and distribute applications.

A number of medical applications are already available [12], an example of which is Medscape, featuring:

- 7000+ drug references;
- 3500+ disease clinical references;
- 2500+ clinical images and procedure videos;
- robust drug interaction tool checker;
- CME activities.

9.6 Summary

In a way, what the technology future holds for teaching and learning depends very much on the kinds of technologies available and how educators and audiences embrace technology and use it in innovative ways to inform and deliver education, training, assessment, feedback etc. In terms of what the future holds, it is good to look back at individual technologies and media such as voice, sound, vision, animation, robotics, electronic control and interfacing via computers. While each of these technologies and media has brought individual products to market, a really powerful teaching and learning context is captured by a holistic approach to these, bringing them together into a focused immersive environment such as a patient simulator.

For future technologies to work effectively to enhance teaching and learning, we look to those entrepreneurs with 'eyes in the sky, feet on the ground', and the past has taught us that the future of technological aids for teaching and learning is hard to predict due to the rapidly changing technology environment.

References

1 Social software. http://en.wikipedia.org/wiki/Social_software.
2 Zebra authoring environment. http://jaycross.posterous.com/michael-allen-describes-the-future-of-authori.
3 Unity game authoring software. http://unity3d.com/unity/.
4 Moore's Law. http://en.wikipedia.org/wiki/Moore%27s_law.

5   Tom Vander Ark. http://www.huffingtonpost.com/tom-vander-ark.

6   Naisbitt J. Megatrends: Ten New Directions Transforming Our Lives. New York, Warner Books, 1982. http://www.huffingtonpost.com/tom-vander-ark/8-megatrends-shaping-the-_b_855010.html.

7   Kuhn B. Technology is a Game Changer for Learning. http://www.shift2future.com/2010/12/technology-is-game-changer-for-learning.html.

8   Touch-screen technology. http://www.youtube.com/watch?v=jbkSRLYSojo&feature=player_embedded#at=260.

9   The Design of Personal Mobile Technologies for Lifelong Learning. http://www.eee.bham.ac.uk/sharplem/Papers/handler%20comped.pdf.

10   Neuro-surgical implant experiments. http://www.kevinwarwick.com/Cyborg2.htm.

11   4G technology. http://www.cyberzest.com/4g-and-the-future-of-mobile-technology-part-1/.

12   Mobile medical apps reviews and commentary. http://www.imedicalapps.com/2011/01/top-free-android-medical-apps-healthcare-professionals/.

[All links last accessed on 30 September 2011.]

Chapter 10 **Conclusion**

During the period 2000 to 2010, it could be argued that e-learning has 'come of age'; from the early days where advances in technology (particularly desktop computing) drove learning developments that focused on the technology rather than the learning, to the opposite where technology facilitates learning and appropriate media are utilised to fit the learning requirement.

During the same period, much educational research was produced and it is not difficult now to find a large body of evidence that shows that 'e-learning works'; indeed, not only has it been shown to work, but evidence shows that learning outcomes are as good as those delivered by other learning methods.

For teachers and learners, technology-enhanced solutions provide unique opportunities and the chapters on using them to learn and teach explore these, providing examples and contexts and highlighting key messages to empower us in our endeavours to provide and engage with pedagogically sound solutions. How often do we feel we wish something were available to join all this up? Perhaps for teachers, using complementary delivery methodologies to deliver learning gives an opportunity to optimise learning. Using more than one method, e.g. face-to-face sessions supported by e-learning opportunities, also addresses learners' individual learning preferences.

There is no doubt that ongoing developments in mobile technologies have provided new and revolutionary ways to deliver and engage with learning. The concept of 'just in time, just enough and on the move' describes quite simply the new opportunities; in busy professional working environments, characterised by the need to work at different levels and switch between these at a moment's notice, multitasking and supporting colleagues, can we

How to Succeed at E-learning, First Edition. Peter Donnelly, Joel Benson, and Paul Kirk.

© 2012 John Wiley & Sons Ltd. Published 2012 by John Wiley & Sons Ltd.

provide appropriately focused information and learning opportunities just in time?

In parallel with learning environments has come the need to integrate assessment with delivery; a key component of learning, asking questions, providing answers and gaining feedback. Bloom's taxonomy of learning informs us about levels of learning and how we can assess learning effectively at the different levels by using appropriately framed questions. Many learning management systems provide us with the tools to host content and deliver it, provide assessment and store the outcomes. The new challenge at the moment is integrating phone technology effectively into these management systems.

Chapter 8 outlines the considerable growth there has been in the number of providers and the number of courses available that lead to e-learning qualifications. Much has been learned by the institutions providing these opportunities and the market continues to grow, fuelled by learners' need to learn flexibly.

Some e-learning contexts are immersive, such as VR and Second Life. Here technology plays a key part in facilitating an 'alternative reality' that can be configured and adapted to imitate real-world scenarios, but excluding the risks associated with reality. If we get it wrong in VR, we can just start again. These are extremely valuable experiences for learners, with opportunities to debrief and use an iterative approach to 'getting it right'.

In deciding whether to provide e-learning opportunities, in modern times we also have to factor in the developmental context of modern learners. At the present time (2011), anyone over 20 years old has grown up through an education system that has used technology in numerous ways to facilitate and enrich the learning experience. It is important to realise, therefore, when we address a learning context that there is considerable expectation that technology will play a significant part; e-learning is not an option, in modern times it is an accepted and expected component.

The challenge to all teachers is therefore to look at the curriculum and plan its delivery, assessment and feedback, including appropriate aims, objectives and learning activities. Sometimes some of this will be done for you – e.g. the assessment part may be a formal examination such as a written exam, case-based discussion or mini clinical evaluation exercise; your role may then be 'How can I optimise learning for these learners?' – a modern approach will mean that more than one delivery method will be used. You may get your learners to attend a face-to-face session with small-group work around a particular objective. In order to support that, perhaps an e-learning component might be a discussion forum led by the tutor prior to the face-to-face. The electronic component will mean that when your learners do the face-to-face session, they will be familiar with some component that was previously discussed online; so you have, by utilising this electronic intervention, changed the nature of the face-to-face and elevated it to a higher level of learning.

The converse is also true – you can do the face-to-face and follow it up with an electronic component. The key message is that you are using more than one approach and blending them to optimise learning.

The various chapters of this book will lead you through many different scenarios, many different media and many ways to use e-learning. It will guide you to help avoid the major pitfalls and provide ideas for ways in which you can enhance your teaching approach. As a learner, you will gain ideas on how you can develop strategies for maximising your potential to learn and, importantly, retain your learning.

Index

How to Succeed at E-learning, First Edition. Peter Donnelly, Joel Benson, and
Paul Kirk.

© 2012 John Wiley & Sons Ltd. Published 2012 by John Wiley & Sons Ltd.